Why Dogs *Can't Eat* Chocolate

Why Dogs

— Can't Eat —

Chocolate

How Medicines Work and How
YOU Can Take Them Safely

Dr. Louise Achey

NEW YORK

Why Dogs *Can't Eat* Chocolate
How Medicines Work and How YOU Can Take Them Safely

Published in New York, New York, by Morgan James Publishing. Morgan James and The Entrepreneurial Publisher are trademarks of Morgan James, LLC. www.MorganJamesPublishing.com

The Morgan James Speakers Group can bring authors to your live event. For more information or to book an event visit The Morgan James Speakers Group at www.TheMorganJamesSpeakersGroup.com.

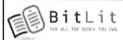

FREE eBook edition for your existing eReader with purchase

PRINT NAME ABOVE

For more information, instructions, restrictions, and to register your copy, go to **www.bitlit.ca/readers/register** or use your QR Reader to scan the barcode:

ISBN 978-1-61448-967-2 paperback
ISBN 978-1-61448-968-9 eBook
ISBN 978-1-61448-969-6 audio
ISBN 978-1-61448-970-2 hardcover
Library of Congress Control Number:
2013952367

Cover design by Alece Birnbach
Cartoons by Alece Birnbach
Notes illustration by Vince Palko
Other illustrations by the author

Quantity discounts are available to your company, educational institution or organization for educational purposes, gifts or fundraising.
Contact Dr. Louise Achey at (509) 658-2570
P.O. Box 98, Naches, WA 98937
www.AskDrLouise.com

In an effort to support local communities, raise awareness and funds, Morgan James Publishing donates a percentage of all book sales for the life of each book to Habitat for Humanity Peninsula and Greater Williamsburg.

Get involved today, visit
www.MorganJamesBuilds.com.

Habitat for Humanity®
Peninsula and
Greater Williamsburg
Building Partner

Disclaimer

All of the information in this book is intended to supplement and support the advice of your medical care professional, not to contradict or conflict with it.

Please, please DO NOT stop any of your prescription medicines without first consulting a medical professional!

Your results and responses may vary from those of others and should be monitored by you working together with your medical care provider.

Dedication

To my pharmacist colleagues,
who devote their professional lives
to helping people take medicine safely -
Applying their knowledge, experience,
and skill to assure optimal drug therapy outcomes
for the patients we serve

and

the Institute for Safe Medication Practices (ISMP),
making the prevention of medication errors
its primary mission for over 30 years.

Contents

Acknowledgements

Thank you to Bill Hayton, Ph.D. for introducing me to and inspiring me to explore the world of pharmacodynamics (WHICH medicine) and pharmacokinetics (HOW MUCH medicine). I really appreciate your allowing me as a pharmacy student to collaborate with you in publishing your lecture notes in our campus bookstore, because there weren't any textbooks written yet about those topics.

A very special thank you to Dr. Ahna Brutlag, DVM, veterinary toxicologist and Assistant Director of Veterinary Services at Pet Poison Helpline (www.petpoisonhelpline.com) for reviewing the information about theobromine toxicity in Chapter 1, The Dark Side of Chocolate, for accuracy.

With deep appreciation to Linda K. Porlier who gave me idea for the book title and the guidance to get it published. Linda knew just when to push and when to back off, and her assistance with editing has been priceless.

And to my husband Charlie, whose encouragement made this all possible. You're the greatest!

Preface

In February of 1980 I joined the pharmacy staff of Samaritan Hospital, a 50-bed hospital in Moses Lake, Washington. While there I discovered Michael Cohen's bi-monthly column in the publication *Hospital Pharmacy*. Each of Michael's columns described a specific medication error and gave practical suggestions on how we could prevent them from happening in our own institution.

Twenty-three years later, Michael Cohen is still writing that column and continuing the vital work of reducing medication errors and their dangerous, potentially tragic consequences.

In 1990, Michael Cohen and Neil Davis founded the nonprofit Institute for Safe Medication Practices (ISMP), with its mission *"turning errors into education"*. The ISMP continues that mission today, providing impartial, timely and accurate information on how to prevent medication errors in hospitals and other medical settings.

If you have ever sought treatment at an ER or have been hospitalized, then you have benefited from the efforts of the ISMP to reduce your risk of having a medical professional give you the wrong medicine or the wrong dose.

A percentage from the sale of each book of **Why Dogs Can't Eat Chocolate** will be donated to the Institute for Safe Medicine Practices Foundation to support their important work in making medication prescribing, dispensing and administration safer for all of us.

Introduction

This book was written to help you keep your dog safe from poisoning from chocolate AND to help you understand what your doctor and pharmacist want you to know about how to take medicine safely. According to the Institute of Medicine, at least 1.5 million *preventable* adverse medication events occur every year.[1]

A recent report from the Centers for Disease Control and Prevention (CDC) shows more Americans die from accidental overdoses of prescription medicines than are killed in motor vehicle accidents.[2]

Using the example of how dogs can die from eating something that's quite harmless to you, I'll show you HOW and WHY medicines work, how TOO MUCH medicine and medication mishaps can happen, and how to prevent medication mishaps from happening to you or a loved one.

When you understand how TOO MUCH medicine happens and how to avoid it, you can better take advantage of all the information about how to take your medicine from your doctor, pharmacist and available on the Internet. That's because you'll see *how it relates to YOU*.

With 75% of all visits to a physician resulting in a prescription[3], the American medical care system depends more and more on powerful medicines that are intended to help but have the potential to cause harm.

Medicines are a very powerful yet unpredictable treatment because they don't work the same in everyone. *The book you hold in your hands explains WHY, and exactly WHAT you can do about it.*

Part I of Why Dogs Can't Eat Chocolate tells the story of Barney the baby Basset Hound and why chocolate is so dangerous for dogs, including the actual amount of chocolate that would kill a dog the size of Barney.

In Part II, How Medicines Work I introduce the basic building blocks of how and why medicines do what they do. Chapter 2, *Which Medicine?* explains HOW medicines work and Chapter 3, *How Much Medicine?* shows how TOO MUCH medicine can happen and how dangerous it is to us, just like too much chocolate is dangerous to a dog. The last 3 chapters go into more detail of how medicines move into and out of your body.

Part III, How to Take Medicine Safely introduces the "3 D"s of Drug Therapy and the importance of having each of them included in a current list of all of your medicines that you share with all of your medical care providers.

In Part IV you'll get specific strategies that can dramatically reduce the chances of being harmed by any medication you take. Alece Birnbach's artistic talent makes the 5 Key Strategies for Protecting You and Your Loved Ones From The Dangers of Drug Therapy really come to life.

Additional examples of exactly how you can avoid trouble with your medicines are given in Part V, 25 Ways You Can Avoid Medication Mishaps.

How To Use This Book

This book is organized into 5 sections directly related to its title. It starts with *Why Dogs Can't Eat Chocolate*, covers *How Medicines Work*, and finishes with *How You Can Take Them Safely*. Each section builds on the previous one but **go ahead and skip around** if that works better for you.

As you read, you'll see these 3 icons:

The cat calls your attention to important ideas about how to take your medicines safely.

The dog provides more medical terms and more detail. Feel free to skip these if you don't want or need additional information.

The bone marks important concepts throughout each chapter and highlights a summary at the end of each chapter.

There are also several blank pages labeled Notes where you can write down your ideas about what you are reading. In the back, a Resources section includes blank and downloadable medication lists and smart phone apps to help you keep any list of your medications current.

PART I

Why Dogs
— *Can't Eat* —
Chocolate

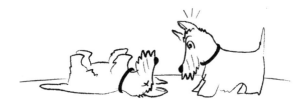

1 Barney's Story

Debra grew up on a farm with dogs the size of golden retrievers and labs, but she'd always wanted a dog of her very own. When she got her first "real job" and moved out on her own, her father drove with her to Oregon to pick up her very own puppy, a Bassett Hound she named Barney.

Barney was a sweetheart of a dog. From the time she brought him home as a puppy, he made all of Debra's friends and family laugh just being around him. Bassett Hounds are born with their ears almost full-grown, which drag on the ground until they grow into them. Debra and Barney loved to drive up to her family's cabin in the mountains and go on winter walks, his big floppy ears dragging along in the snow at her side as he looked up at her. So cute!

Barney loved to chase the farm cats around, just for fun, and his favorite toy was an old half-chewed tennis ball he liked to chase after when anyone would throw it for him. Although he was just a little guy, Barney had a big Bassett Hound "bay-bark."' When Debra arrived home after work or an errand he would show her how glad he was by standing up and giving her a big happy " AAARRRFFF, AAARRRFFF, AAARRRFFF, AAARRRFFF!" which was music to her ears.

It was late summer in 1974 when Debra headed up to the mountains to meet up with some friends from Seattle to go camping over the weekend. When she couldn't locate them, she drove instead to her grandmother's house in Harrah, Washington to spend the night with her.

On the way she stopped at a local Woolworth's store to pick up some snacks for the trip, including a bag of chocolate stars, her favorite. At 19 months old, Barney was small for a Bassett, weighing only 18 pounds. He loved to ride in the front passenger seat of Debra's 1971 white Ford Pinto Runabout, where he could stand on his hind legs to look for cats and his favorite target, COWS. As they pulled out of her driveway, she smiled as he pressed his nose against the window, scanning for cats and COWS to bark at.

Turning onto I-82 at Ellensburg, a movement at her right caught Debra's attention. The sound of sniffing was followed by the sound of crinkling paper as Barney found the chocolate stars she'd stashed on the floor.

He really seemed to enjoy the candy, and before she realized it he'd finished off the entire bag. As she came up on the freeway exit to her grandmother's farm, she wondered, could eating all of that candy make Barney sick?

Surely he would be fine, she reasoned. Her family's farm dogs had eaten chocolate candy from time to time, without any ill effects. Barney acted just like himself when they arrived, chasing after the farm cats, his floppy ears flying.

Because her grandmother wouldn't allow dogs in the house, Debra settled Barney in the fenced back yard instead. But when she checked on him the next morning it was obvious that something was wrong. There was diarrhea all over the back yard, and when she called his name he acted listless. Poor Barney! He couldn't settle enough to eat or sleep, and kept having explosive diarrhea.

Debra called the closest veterinarian open on Saturday and took Barney in just as soon as they opened. The vet gave him fluids and told her it was most likely an insecticide poisoning from farm chemicals, but that didn't make sense, as Debra's family had always been meticulously careful about handling and storing chemicals.

On Sunday Debra had to get back to work and picked Barney up from the vet clinic by her grandmother's and drove the 3 hours home. Monday morning he was still restless and vomiting, and Debra took him to another veterinarian, hoping for a second opinion.

She told the second vet what the first one had suggested, and how she doubted that Barney had come in contact with any farm or garden chemicals. The second vet shook his head, told her it looked just like poisoning and tried his best to administer fluids and supportive care.

Sadly, little Barney didn't get better. He started having seizures that evening and died the next day.

The Dark Side of Chocolate

Why did Barney die?

How could chocolate, enjoyed by humans all over the world be so dangerous to Debra's little buddy, Barney?

and

Why is chocolate dangerous to our dogs *but not to us?*

In Barney's body, the chocolate stars he ate acted like poison.

When given a medicine, humans and animals first react or respond to it, then they detoxify and remove it. Although dogs respond to and detoxify most medicines just like humans do, there are some important exceptions.

One of these medicines is theobromine, found in chocolate.

Many medicines work exactly the same in dogs as they do in humans, but there are some that do not. With chocolate, that difference can be FATAL!

Chocolate is made from roasting the seeds of the *theobroma cacao* tree. Its name is a combination of the Greek word theobroma, which means "food of the gods", and its Aztec name, the cacao tree.

For humans, eating chocolate may be more than just tasty; it may have health benefits as well. Roasted cacao seeds (beans) contain flavanols, which are natural compounds found in many fruits and vegetables.

Flavanols are desirable because they are associated with a decreased risk of heart disease. In general, the higher the amount of cacao in a particular chocolate product, the "darker" the chocolate is and the higher the amount of flavanols it will contain. This has led to an increase in the popularity and availability of candy and baked goods containing dark chocolate.

Flavanols are not the only compounds produced by the cacao tree. Theobromine and caffeine are naturally occurring stimulants found in the cacao bean and its outer shell.

To make chocolate, cacao beans are first picked, cured, and then roasted. The heat from the roasting process drives most of the theobromine from the cacao bean into its outer shell and splits it open to expose the valuable inner bean inside.

After roasting, discarded cacao shells were originally recycled by adding them to animal feed. Tragically, this practice caused deaths in young horses, calves, piglets, chickens and ducks. Upon investigation, the deaths were determined to be from eating toxic concentrations of theobromine from the cacao shells. Today, recycling of cacao shells is limited to use in landscape mulch.

Theobromine and caffeine are not concentrated enough in chocolate to affect humans, but in high concentrations can be toxic to small animals.

Although most of the theobromine originally contained in the cacao bean is removed during the roasting process, there still remains enough of it to sicken and kill many small animals if they eat enough chocolate.

Caffeine and theobromine are members of a group of naturally occurring compounds called methylxanthines. They are closely related to each other and to theophylline, another methylxanthine found in the leaves of tea plants.

Methylxanthines have been used in stimulant beverages for hundreds of years and in human medicine for decades.

Theobromine and theophylline have been used in humans to treat asthma. They work to relax the airways leading into the lungs, easing chest tightness and relieving wheezing and shortness of breath in those who suffer from asthma.

Caffeine increases mental alertness, improves reaction time, and has been used to treat migraine headaches.

How much chocolate does it take to poison a dog?

The amount of chocolate that is poisonous to a dog depends on three things:

1. The amount of theobromine contained in the chocolate
2. How much chocolate is eaten
3. The size and health of the dog

How much theobromine is found in chocolate?

Theobromine is a component of cacao. The DARKER the chocolate, the higher the concentration of cacao it has and the more theobromine it will contain. The highest concentration of cacao is found in baking chocolate and cocoa powder, shown in Table 1.

Table 1. Cacao Content Comparison[4]

Product	Cacao Content
Baker's® Unsweetened Squares	100%
Hershey's® Cocoa Powder (Original and Special Dark)	100%
Natural Dark Chocolate Bar Endangered Species®	88%
Hershey's® Extra Dark	60%
Ghirardelli® Premium Baking Bar	60%
Hershey's® Special Dark	45%
Nestle® Semi-Sweet Morsels	47%
Hershey's® Milk Chocolate	11%

How much theobromine is fatal to a dog?

The lethal dose of theobromine for a dog is approximately 100-200 mg/kilogram (kg). For an 18-lb (8 kg) dog the same size as Barney, 800 mg of theobromine would be deadly.

 For a dog the size of Barney, eating one 6-ounce bag of semi-sweet chocolate chips or 2 squares of baking chocolate would be dangerous, even fatal.

Table 2 shows the amount and type of chocolate that would contain 800mg theobromine, a lethal dose for a dog the size of little Barney.

Table 2. Theobromine Content of Chocolate[4]

Product	% Cacao	Theobromine per ounce	* 800mg Theobromine
Baker's® Unsweetened Squares	100%	390-450 mg	2 oz.
Cocoa Powder	100%	400-737 mg	8 Tbsp (1/2 cup)
Ghirardelli® Premium Baking Bar	60%	330 mg	2.5 oz.
Semisweet and Sweet Dark Chocolate	45-70%	130-150 mg	6 oz.
Nestle® Semi-Sweet Morsels	47%	125 mg	6 oz.
Hershey's® Milk Chocolate	11%	40 mg	20 oz.

* Lethal dose for a Barney-sized dog (18 lb or 8 kg)

> If you suspect your dog has eaten chocolate, collect the container or wrappers and contact your veterinarian or a pet poison control center immediately.

Both national pet poison control centers charge a fee to provide veterinary advice over the phone. Be prepared with a credit card before you call. Follow up calls are included in the fee.

Pet Poison Centers

- Pet Poison Helpline
  (800) 213-6680
  www.petpoisonhelpline.com

- ASPCA Animal Poison Information Center
  (888) 426-4435
  www.aspca.org/pet-care/poison-control/

There are also regional poison centers that may also be of assistance with an animal poisoning. Check with your local poison center for more information. If you call (800) 222-1222, you will be connected to the Poison Center nearest you.

Is theobromine only toxic to dogs?

Theobromine is not just poisonous to dogs. Any small animal is at risk. Cats are picky and usually avoid chocolate, but dogs love the smell and taste of chocolate and will enthusiastically eat it. Small dogs will readily eat enough chocolate to consume a lethal dose of theobromine.

What effect does theobromine have on a dog?

Dogs are unable to detoxify theobromine easily. Too much theobromine can cause a racing heart, abnormal heart rhythms, vomiting, diarrhea, tremors, seizures and collapse.

Mild stomach upset is associated with a less serious poisoning and with treatment the chance of recovery is very good.

Elevated heart rates, abnormal heart rhythms, tremors and seizures are signs of serious theobromine toxicity and even with treatment the likelihood of recovery is much lower.

If chocolate can kill a pet, why aren't small children at risk from chocolate poisoning?

Small children are not at risk for poisoning from theobromine in chocolate because humans are able to rapidly detoxify it. A human can detoxify theobromine twice as quickly as a dog.

Theobromine is not the only danger that lurks in chocolate. The high fat content of chocolate can trigger painful and life-threatening pancreatitis, an inflammation of the pancreas.

For more information, ask your veterinarian about high fat foods and your pet.

- Dogs can detoxify many medicines just like humans do. Veterinarians treat dogs with some of the same medicines that doctors use to treat humans.

- Humans and dogs respond differently to detoxifying some medicines. One of these medicines is theobromine, found in chocolate.

- The darker and more concentrated the chocolate, the more theobromine it will contain. The most concentrated chocolate is found in cocoa powder and cocoa squares used for baking.

- Dogs love the taste and smell of chocolate and will readily eat enough to cause a fatal poisoning from theobromine.

- Small children are not at risk of poisoning from chocolate because humans detoxify theobromine twice as quickly as dogs.

- The smaller the dog, the less chocolate they can tolerate. For an 18-pound dog like Barney, one 6-ounce bag of semi-sweet chocolate chips is enough to cause death from theobromine poisoning.

- If you suspect your dog has eaten chocolate, collect the container or wrappers and contact your veterinarian immediately. You can also call one of the special poison centers for pets. The Resources section in the Appendix of this book has pet poison control center contact information.

- Chocolate has a high fat content that can trigger painful and life-threatening pancreatitis in your dog.

Notes

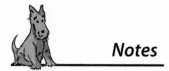

Notes

PART II

How Medicines Work

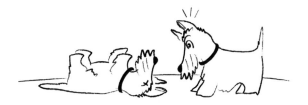

2 WHICH Medicine?

What makes something useful as a medicine?

A medicine is used to treat a particular condition because it can CHANGE something in your body that will help you get better.

What's the difference between a medicine your doctor prescribes to lower your high blood pressure and a medicine you take to relieve your headache?

The difference between these 2 medicines is what they CHANGE in your body. If you have an infection, an antibiotic can help your body fight the infection by attacking the organism that is infecting you. If you have a headache, a pain reliever can relieve your discomfort by blocking your pain.

17

HOW do medicines do what they do?

Medicines work by creating a CHANGE in your body. They do this by attaching to a special place which then causes a change in your body.

Medicines are like KEYS. They "fit" into any place in your body with a particular shape that matches with the way they are shaped and when they do it usually triggers a change in your body.

Medicines are like KEYS.

Imagine walking up to a bank vault with a thick glass door. There are shelves from floor to ceiling packed with chests and boxes of varying sizes and shapes, each of them locked securely with a padlock. Each padlock is a little different. Some are very simple, others are ornate, and they come in sizes from as large as your fist to the size of your pinkie finger.

Hanging on a hook just to the left of the vault door is a round key ring as big as a salad plate, packed with keys of varied sizes. Picking it up with your left hand, you push open the door with your right and step into the vault, the thick glass door softly whooshing shut behind you. Each chest's padlock is labeled, and most of them have at least one key labeled to match.

The chest in front of you has several keys corresponding to it, so you pick one and try it out. It doesn't quite fit. With 4 other keys marked as belonging to that lock, you pick another one to try. It fits all the way in and turns, but the pad-lock doesn't open. Pulling that key out, you select a third key, insert it, and as you turn it the lock pops open in your hand.

Each of the keys on your key ring represent a different medicine, and the padlocks represent where they could "fit" in your body.

Medicines are like KEYS.

Medicines "work" if they can fit into a shaped area in your body, like a key fitting into a lock. WHICH shape of lock a medicine can "fit" into and WHERE these "locks" are in your body will determine WHAT TYPE of change happens when you take it.

When a medicine "fits into" to a certain spot, it "sticks", or binds to it. The place that a medicine can "stick" or bind to is called a receptor because it "receives" the medicine, like a key going into a lock.

Both the medicine and its receptor have to be shaped in a way that allows the medicine to attach to it, similar to how the two sides of Velcro® stick together, how a key fits into a lock, or how one puzzle piece fits into the one right next to it.

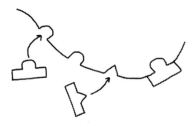

Figure 1. Medicine Binding To a Receptor

When a medicine finds and binds to its receptor, it triggers a predictable change in your body. For example, a blood pressure medicine binds to a different receptor than a pain medicine and causes a different effect on your body.

Medicines can bind only to places shaped in a way that allows them to "fit". This limits them to specific receptors, like a key will only fit certain types of locks. Some receptors are very specialized, and others are more general. Medicines that can bind to more specialized receptors will cause a more focused change than those that bind to more general receptors.

The more specific and focused the receptors your medicine binds to, the less likely you are to experience unintended or undesirable changes, called side effects. Side effects can range from minor annoyances to severe debilitating symptoms that can completely overwhelm any potential benefit you might receive from the medicine.

The best medicine for you will cause only a very specific and focused change in your body that matches what you and your doctor expect from it.

How does a doctor choose a medicine?

A medicine is chosen by how it works. Medicines are organized into groups that do similar things in your body, called therapeutic classes. Examples of some therapeutic classes are antibiotics, analgesics (pain relievers), and antihypertensive agents (medicines that lower blood pressure).

REMEMBER

Inside each therapeutic group of medicines are smaller groups that bind to the same or to similar receptors. These smaller groups of related medicines are called medication classes or drug classes.

Medicines of the same drug class create similar responses by binding to the same receptor and are used for the same reasons. The reason a medicine is used is also called its indication.

WHICH Medicine?

To treat an infection caused by bacteria, you need something that can kill bacteria: an antibiotic. Antibiotics are a group of medicines that contain several drug classes, including penicillins, sulfa drugs, and cephalosporins. Each class binds to a different spot (receptor) on certain bacteria.

Medicines that bind to the same receptor have the same action and are grouped in the same drug class. For example, the penicillin drug class has several related penicillin medicines that fit onto the same receptor and create the same killing effect on certain types of bacteria.

After binding to their receptor, most medicines will trigger a fairly predictable change in your body. This is also called *activating* the receptor. Some medicines, however, DON'T activate their receptor. When these medicines bind to their receptors, nothing happens. It's like putting a key into the ignition of your car but when you turn the key the car doesn't start.

Why would a doctor use a medicine that doesn't change anything when it binds to its receptor?

Sometimes we can change something in the body by blocking the action of a medicine that can do the opposite type of effect. We can use one medication to block the action of another medicine by covering up its receptor, similar to someone inserting a key into a padlock. If a lock already has a key sitting in it, you can't put another key in there at the same time!

A medicine can't bind to its receptor if another medicine is there first, covering it up.

Medicines that can block receptors but will not cause any direct change are called antagonists. They work by preventing the change the other medicine could create *IF* it was able to bind to that receptor.

How a medicine works is called its "mechanism of action" or MOA and is determined by which receptor it binds to in your body.

The MOA of a medicine determines what it is used for, also known as its therapeutic indication.

Before a medicine can be marketed and sold in the United States, it has to meet certain standards of safety and effectiveness set by the Food and Drug Administration (FDA). The FDA is responsible for approving which diseases or medical conditions a medicine can be marketed for.

A medicine can have more than one approved indication from the FDA, and doctors are not limited to prescribing medications only for FDA approved indications. Prescribing a medicine outside its FDA approved medical conditions is called "off-label" use.

- A medicine is used because it DOES SOMETHING to your body. It CHANGES SOMETHING.

- In order for a medicine to DO what it DOES, two things have to happen: it has to bind to a receptor somewhere in your body, and once attached to that receptor, it triggers a change.

- Medicines are like keys. They're only able to bind to those receptors that are shaped in a way that allows them to "fit" them, like a key into a lock.

- The more specialized a medicine is, the more focused the changes to your body will be and the less chance you will experience other, unwanted changes called side effects.

- A medicine is chosen by how it works. How it works depends on what receptor it binds to and what type of change is triggered when it binds to it.

- Medicines are organized into groups that do similar things in your body, called therapeutic classes. Inside each therapeutic class are sub-groups of related medicines called drug classes.

- An antagonist is a medication that works to block the action of another medicine by preventing it from binding to its receptor. A medicine can't bind to its target receptor if another medicine gets there first and covers it up.

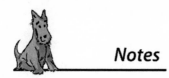

Notes

3

HOW MUCH
Medicine?

How much medicine is the right amount for you?

The best dose of a medicine for you depends on two main things:

- The size of your body
- How fast your body can remove or detoxify the medicine

Taking too little medicine won't provide the desired effect. Taking too much medicine can give you nasty side effects or worse.

With medicines, food supplements, and herbal products, **more is not always better**!

The Center for Disease Control and Prevention (CDC) reports that unintentional overdose of prescription medicine has reached epidemic levels in the United States and is the fastest growing drug problem in our country.

Death from an accidental overdose of prescription medicine is now more common in the United States than being killed in an auto accident!

Body Size and Filling Up Your "Space"

The right dose of medicine for you depends partly on how "large" you are. When it comes to medicine, your body acts like a big container of water. The larger you are, the bigger your container, and the more medicine you will usually need.

As we age, the percentage of water in our body decreases, as shown in Table 3. Going from adult to becoming seniors, our "container" gradually becomes "smaller" and we need less and less medicine.

Table 3. Percent of Water As We Age

Age	% Water as Body Weight
INFANT	75%
ADULT MALE	60%
ADULT FEMALE	50%
SENIOR (>65 YRS)	Decreasing

Another way to say this is: **Fill Up Your Space.**

The amount of medicine you need depends partly on how much is needed to fill your body's container.

The bigger your container, the bigger your "space" and the more medicine you will require. As you age, your container gets smaller and you need less medicine.

Replacing What Your Body Removes

How much medicine is best for you will depend not only on "Filling Up Your Space", but also on how fast your body is removing the medicine.

The best dose of medicine for you is one that balances the amount you are taking (going IN) with the amount that your body is removing (going OUT).

Taking in less medicine in than your body is removing will decrease the amount of medicine in your body and its effects will "wear off".

Taking more medicine than your body can remove will increase the level of medicine in your body, leading to side effects and overdose.

 Most accidental overdoses of prescription medicines are not the result of taking one big dose, but from taking multiple doses too close together.

Instead of just replacing what is being removed, taking doses of a medicine too frequently causes it to build up or accumulate in your body to toxic, potentially fatal levels.

The ability of your body to detoxify and remove medicines is very important. As you age, your body becomes slower at removing medicines and you need less medicine. Alcoholic beverages can also impair your ability to remove certain medicines, causing an exaggerated effect or unintended overdose.

The amount of medicine you need depends on how fast your body is able to detoxify and remove it. You need to take in just enough medicine to REPLACE the medicine that your body is removing.

Like the story of Goldilocks and the Three Bears, if you take too little your medicine won't work, but if you take too much you risk an overdose.

How do you figure out HOW MUCH medicine to take?

For a medicine or herbal supplement to work, it has to go to where its receptors are in your body, "fit into" them and trigger a change. How does a medicine do that?

Medicines *MOVE.*

They go INTO, AROUND, and OUT of your body.

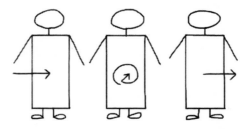

Figure 2. Medicine Goes INTO, AROUND, and OUT of Your Body

In order for a medicine to "work" it has to CHANGE something in your body. To do that, the medicine has to come in contact with a place it can bind to, called a receptor.

First, the medicine gets INSIDE your body. You eat, drink, swallow, rub, inhale, inject or insert it. (I'll explain about this in Chapter 4.)

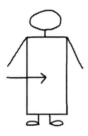

Figure 3. Medicine Goes INTO Your Body

Once the medicine is IN your body, it moves AROUND. (There's more about this in Chapter 5.)

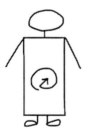

Figure 4. Medicine Moves AROUND In Your Body

As a medicine moves around, whenever it comes in contact with its receptor it binds to it, much like a key into a lock. When enough medicine is binding to its receptors, it will trigger a change in your body.

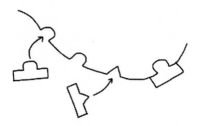

Figure 5. Medicine Binding To Its Receptor

Eventually, medicine goes OUT of your body. As your body removes a medicine there is less and less of it available to bind to its receptor.

As a medicine leaves your body, its effect on you fades away. (In Chapter 6 I explain how medicines and herbal products are removed from your body.)

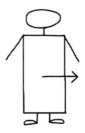

Figure 6. Medicine Goes OUT of Your Body

Some medicines leave your body in the same shape and size as they came in. Other medicines need to be detoxified or changed FIRST before they can be removed.

If you don't get ENOUGH medicine you won't get better, but getting TOO MUCH medicine can be dangerous, even fatal!

In order to get the desired response from a medicine, whether it's lowering your blood pressure, relieving a muscle spasm in your back, or decreasing your "bad" cholesterol, **you need to take enough medicine to bind to the receptors that the medicine fits on, but not so much that you experience an exaggerated effect, side effects or toxicity.**

Doctors and medical professionals do their best to choose the safest, most effective dose of medicine for you, but there is too much variability between people to get it right every time.

No drug works in everyone, and no drug works the same in everyone. Getting the best dose of medicine for you is a process of trial and error.

- For a medicine or herbal supplement to work, it has to go to where its receptors are, bind to them and trigger a change in your body.

- How big you are and how fast your body removes a particular medicine determines the best dose of it for you.

- The right dose of medicine for you is partly related to your size. If you don't have enough medicine binding to its target receptors, you won't notice much effect.

- If your dose of medicine binds to too many receptors, you will experience side effects or toxicity.

- After taking the first dose of your medicine, to keep its beneficial effect going you only need to take enough to REPLACE what your body is able to remove.

- Most fatal accidental overdoses of prescription medicines are not the result of taking one big dose, but from taking multiple doses too close together.

- No drug works in everyone, and no drug works the same in everyone. The receptors or binding places in YOUR body may be shaped differently than that same receptor in other people's bodies.

- Doctors do their best to choose the safest and most effective dose of medicine for you, but because of the variations between people in the shape and quantity of their medicine receptors, it's a process of trial and error.

Notes

4 Medicine Goes IN

For a medicine or herbal supplement to work on you, it has to go to where its receptors are and bind or "fit into" them, which then triggers a change in your body. First of all, it has to get IN.

How do medicines get into your body?

How a medicine is able to get into your body will determine what form it can take.

There are several forms that medicines can take to enter your body:

- A pill or liquid that you swallow (oral)
- A dissolving tablet you place under your tongue (sublingual)
- Into your lungs as you inhale (inhalation)
- Into your nose as a spray (nasal spray)
- Into your lungs as a mist created by a machine (nebulized)

- Applied to your skin as a patch (transdermal)
- Rubbed onto your skin (topical)
- Inserted into your rectum (rectally)
- Inserted into your vagina (vaginally)
- Injected into the layer right under your skin (subcutaneously)
- Injected into your muscle (intramuscularly)
- Injected into your vein (intravenously)

What happens to a medicine after you take it?

After you take a dose of medicine, it goes to work at getting into your body. Another name for this activity is absorption. Absorption is the process of how medicines get into your body.

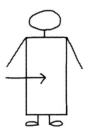

Figure 7. Medicine Goes IN

Most medicines are designed to take by mouth because it is easier and less painful to swallow a pill than to insert or inject it. Another reason that medicines are given as a pill or tablet if at all possible is that liquid medicines made into injections tend to disintegrate more quickly over time than solid medicines.

When you swallow a liquid, tablet or capsule, your stomach is its next stop.

Unless protected by a special coating, most pills and capsules will start dissolving immediately when they arrive in your stomach. They'll mix with any food, liquids or gastric juices in there. Chewable tablets, "melting" tablets designed to dissolve on your tongue and liquid medicine will start working a few minutes earlier than tablets or capsules because they do not have to take the time to dissolve first.

Once a medicine dissolves in your stomach, it needs to get into your bloodstream in order to find and bind to its target receptors.

Most medicines move into your blood from your small intestine instead of from your stomach. Your stomach empties its contents directly into your small intestine, where the mix of fluids, gastric juices, dissolved medicines and any partially digested food flow along together toward your large intestine and colon.

There are lots of blood vessels lining your small intestine that work to move dissolved medicines out of your small intestine and into your bloodstream where they are carried by your blood throughout your body. This process is called absorption.

Once in your bloodstream, a medicine travels throughout your body, where it eventually finds its receptors, binds to them, and triggers the change it's responsible for creating.

How a medicine is able to get into your body will determine what form it can take.

Swallowing a tablet or capsule is not the only way to take a medicine, although it's the most common and least expensive way.

Some medicines can be absorbed from your skin right into your bloodstream, allowing them to be given transdermally as patches. Some medication patches are applied daily; others are applied less frequently, either every 3 days, twice a week, or weekly.

There are some medicines that can enter the bloodstream when inserted into the rectum or vagina. The medicine is mixed with another substance that melts at body temperature, then formed into a bullet-shaped suppository. A suppository is designed to melt at body temperature in order for the liquefied medicine to move directly into your bloodstream through the lining of your rectum or vagina.

How much of each dose of medicine gets all the way into your body?

When you swallow a pill, there's no guarantee the entire amount of medicine in it will get into your bloodstream. Sometimes part or all of a medicine will be destroyed in the stomach or left behind in the small intestine.

Any medicine that doesn't get transported into your bloodstream as it moves through your small intestine continues moving through the rest of your digestive tract along with any partially digested food and digestive juices, eventually coming out in your feces through a bowel movement.

How do you "lose" part of a dose of medicine?

With some medicines, if you have food in your stomach when you swallow it, some of the medicine can combine with some of your food particles instead of dissolving completely. This can keep some of the medicine from being absorbed into your bloodstream, causing less effect or even treatment failure.

Some medicines are best taken without food in your stomach to ensure good absorption. That means avoiding food for at least one hour before or for at least 2 hours after any meal.

How much medicine gets into your bloodstream is called its bioavailability.

100% bioavailability means that ALL of the medicine in the tablet or capsule you have taken has moved into your bloodstream and is now in your body, moving around and able to bind to any of its receptors it comes in contact with.

50% bioavailability means that only half of the medicine you have taken is now in your bloodstream. The rest of it didn't make it out of your intestine; instead, it's carried along through your digestive tract and eventually removed in your feces.

Some medicines are affected by direct contact with certain minerals. Calcium, iron and magnesium can actually attach themselves to certain medicine molecules, physically changing them and preventing them from being absorbed into your body.

If you take one of these types of medicines, you should avoid taking supplements and vitamins that contain these minerals for 2 hours before and 2 or 3 hours after taking this kind of medicine.

Some medicines can't be taken by mouth because they are completely destroyed by the normal digestive juices of your stomach.

Other medicines are physically too big to be able to move across the wall of your small intestine into your bloodstream.

Medicines that cannot be absorbed as a pill or tablet may instead need to be given as an injection or a skin patch. Insulin is an example of a medicine that needs to be injected instead of taken as a pill.

Despite special treatment, some medicines STILL aren't absorbed very well. One example of this is alendronate, originally the brand name

Fosamax®, which is a tablet taken once daily or once weekly to strengthen weak or thin bones. Even under the best conditions, only about 3% of the alendronate in each tablet gets into the bloodstream, the rest staying behind in the small intestine and then eliminated through the feces.

REMEMBER

- For a medicine or herbal supplement to work, it has to go to where its receptors are, bind or "fit into" them and trigger a change in your body. To do that, it first has to get INTO your body, usually by getting into your bloodstream.

- Absorption is the process of how medicines get into your bloodstream.

- Once a medicine gets into your bloodstream it is carried throughout your body.

- How a medicine is able to get into your bloodstream will determine what form it takes, for example: tablet, patch, inhaler, suppository or injection.

- Most medicines are given by mouth as a liquid, tablet, or capsule because it is less expensive and less painful to take a medicine by swallowing it than to have to inject it or insert it.

- In order for medicine in a pill or tablet to completely dissolve and move from your small intestine into your bloodstream it may be best to take it without any food in your stomach.

- Some medicines cannot get into your bloodstream from your small intestine because they are either destroyed by digestive juices in your stomach or are physically too big to move through the lining of your small intestine.

Notes

5 Medicine Moves AROUND

What happens after a medicine gets into your bloodstream?

Once a medicine enters your body and gets into your bloodstream, it needs to find and bind to its target receptor so it can trigger the change it is designed to do.

You need enough medicine in the right place to be binding to its target receptors in order to trigger the change you want to have happen.

If enough medicine binds to its target receptors, then:

- If you're taking a pain medicine, your headache eases.
- If you're taking a medicine for nausea, your vomiting stops.
- If you're taking an antibiotic, your infection improves.

How much medicine do you need?

You need enough medicine so that it can bind to the "best" number of receptors in your body.

Enough to **FILL UP YOUR SPACE.**

If you think of yourself as a hollow container like an empty gas tank, the bigger your tank, the more gasoline it will take to "fill it up". The larger your container, the larger the amount or higher the "dose" of medicine you need to "fill it up".

ACTIVITY: The Glass Pitchers

Supplies: 3 Glass containers
              Liquid food Coloring

- Set out 3 empty glass pitchers on a counter or table. Use one small, one medium and one large to represent the relative sizes of an infant, a child, and a large adult.
- Add ¼ cup of water to the smallest glass container, to represent an infant. Add 1 cup of water to the medium glass container to represent a child, and pour 2-4 cups of water into your largest glass container to represent an adult.
- Using 2 cups of water would approximate a small or frail elderly adult, 3 cups of water an average adult, and 4 cups of water would represent a large adult.
- If you don't have glass pitchers, you can substitute 3 clear beverage glasses: small, medium and large.

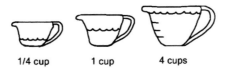

1/4 cup   1 cup   4 cups

Figure 8. Pitchers With Water

- Select a color of liquid food coloring (the darker the better) and put just ONE DROP of it into each glass container. The darker the color you use, the easier it will show up and the better you can see the differences in each of the pitchers.

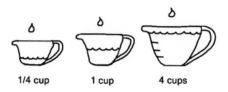

1/4 cup   1 cup   4 cups

Figure 9. Adding Food Coloring To Pitchers

- Now, stir each container with a spoon to mix the coloring throughout. Which container has the darkest liquid, and which one has the lightest? Why?

The color of the water of the smallest container will be much darker than the water in the largest container.

You can see a video demonstration of this at www.AskDrLouise.com.

The larger the container, the more it will dilute the "dose" of food coloring.

Now imagine your body as a hollow container filled with liquid like the water in your glass pitchers. The single drop of food coloring represents a single "dose" of medicine.

The larger your body's container, the more it will dilute a "dose" of medicine.

What's the "best" dose of medicine for you?

In order to prescribe the "best" dose of medicine for you, your doctor tailors the dose to your size. This is why toddlers and most companion animals need less medicine than adults and why just a few pills out of grandma's medicine bottle can be a life-threatening poisoning for a grandchild or beloved pet.

Making sure your dose of medicine is matched to you is very, very important. If you are small, you will **usually** need less medicine than if you are large.

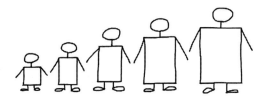

**Figure 10. Different Sizes of
People Need Different Doses**

The best dose of medicine for you is one that "Fills Up" your space, or the container of your body.

 If you don't get ENOUGH medicine you won't get better, but getting TOO MUCH medicine can be dangerous, even fatal!

- You need the right amount of a medicine in your body binding to its target receptors in order to trigger its intended effect.
- If you don't have enough medicine in your body binding to its target receptors, it won't work and you won't notice any improvement.

- If there's too much medicine in your body binding to its target receptors, you'll experience uncomfortable side effects with dangerous, possibly fatal results.

- If you imagine your body as a hollow container filled with water, HOW MUCH medicine you need depends on how much it will take to "Fill Up The Space" of your container.

- When it comes to the right dose of medicine, size matters. Young children and frail seniors usually need less medicine than most adults.

- The best dose of medicine for you is one that will "Fill Up Your Space".

- Making sure your dose of medicine is matched to you is critically important to avoid under-dosing and overdosing.

Notes

6

Medicine Goes OUT

How does a medicine STOP working?

What happens after a medicine enters your body, gets into your bloodstream, moves around, finds its receptor and binds to it, triggering the desired change in your body?

Your body has to detoxify and remove it.

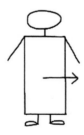

Figure 11. Drug Goes Out

The ability of your body to detoxify and move medicine OUT is the most critically important part of being able to take medicine safely!

 Just like with Debra's puppy Barney, when too much medicine gets IN for your body to be able to detoxify and move OUT, the excess can build up to dangerous, even fatal levels.

A medicine stops working when it can't bind to its target receptor.

Because a medicine works by binding to a receptor to trigger a change, when it can't bind to its receptor, it stops working.

There are two ways your body can stop a medicine from binding to its target receptor:

1. *Eliminating it* by removing it from your bloodstream and body.
2. *Detoxifying it* by changing it so that it no longer fits on its receptor.

Your kidneys and liver have important roles in detoxifying and eliminating medicines from your body.

How Your Kidneys Remove Medicine

Your body eliminates medicine by moving it from your bloodstream into your kidneys and urine, and out of your body when you urinate.

Many medicines are "active", or able to bind to their receptors until your kidneys can physically remove them from your bloodstream.

Removing a medicine directly out of your bloodstream through your kidneys and into your urine makes it stop working because it is now OUT of your body completely and far away from any of its receptors.

ACTIVITY: Fun With Funnels

Supplies: 2 Funnels (1 larger than the other)

- Find 2 funnels, one with a larger outlet on its bottom than the other, if possible.
- Bring your funnels to a sink and pour water into them, one at a time. Notice how the one with the smaller outlet takes longer to empty than the one with the larger outlet?
- With your finger, partly block the bottom of each funnel. How does this change how fast the funnel empties?

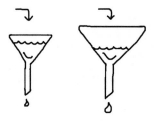

Figure 12. Small and Large Funnels

The funnels emptying out the water is like your kidneys removing medicine from your body by putting it into your urine. The bigger the "funnel", the faster your kidneys can remove a medicine from your body.

After age 35, the ability of your kidneys to remove medicine from your body begins to decrease by about 10% each decade. This is like having the outlet of your funnel gradually get smaller and smaller over time. As you get older, your body will move medicines out of your body more slowly.

Diabetes and high blood pressure can damage your kidneys, making them less able to remove medicine, like partly blocking the funnel's outlet.

 By age 75 your kidneys have lost nearly 40% of their ability to remove medicines from your body, which can cause you problems with taking medicine safely.

How Your Liver Removes Medicine

Your liver is responsible for detoxifying medicine by changing its shape so it no longer fits on or binds to its receptor. Once this happens, the medicine stops working and its effect on your body fades away unless the medicine's new shape can fit on to another receptor.

Changing a potent medicine into a harmless compound by changing its shape is usually done inside your liver. This VERY important process is called biotransformation or detoxification.

Inside your liver are special groups of proteins called liver enzymes that are responsible for rearranging the shapes of many different kinds of molecules.

Your liver enzymes can attach themselves to certain shapes of molecules and take them apart, rearranging their shape. After being reshaped, many medicines or poisons are no longer able to act on our body.

Liver enzymes are critically important to taking medicine safely because we need them to detoxify many different medicines and poisons.

Without certain liver enzymes, you can't detoxify and remove particular medicines and poisons from your body.

Unfortunately, not everyone gets a complete set of these vitally important and specialized liver proteins. There are variants in some liver enzymes documented in certain ethnic populations. Some individuals, families and ethnic groups may completely lack certain liver enzymes. Certain groups of people may have enzymes that are "faster" or "slower" than those found in the general population.

People who have fewer, "slower", or less efficient liver enzymes are likely to experience MORE effects from a medicine than expected. If you detoxify a medicine slowly, it accumulates in your bloodstream, causing serious and potentially dangerous side effects and toxicity.

Those who have liver enzymes that are "faster" or more efficient can detoxify medicine more quickly.

Medicines that are changed or detoxified more rapidly will have less effect on you because their concentration in your body diminishes more quickly, causing their desired effect to "wear off" sooner.

Because each of us is different in how fast we can detoxify medicines, it's VERY important NOT to share your medicines with others!

ACTIVITY: More Fun With Funnels

Supplies: 2 Funnels (1 larger than the other)
            Several glass marbles

- Pour water through each funnel. How fast does the water go out
  the bottom of the larger funnel, compared to the smaller one?
- Your smaller funnel represents people with "slow" liver enzymes
  and your larger funnel ones with "fast" liver enzymes.

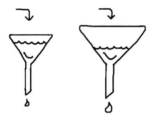

Figure 13. Slow and Fast Liver Enzymes

Whenever the amount of a medicine going
INTO your body exceeds the ability of your liver
enzymes to move it OUT by transforming or
detoxifying it, a dangerous, potentially deadly
accumulation of medicine can occur.

An extremely dangerous situation can occur
when you take in more medicine than your liver
has the enzyme capacity to detoxify it.

When you take in more medicine than your liver enzymes can keep up with, the amount of medicine in your bloodstream can build up to dangerous levels.

The main reason why dogs can't safely eat chocolate is the difference between their liver enzymes and ours.

Our liver can easily detoxify theobromine, while a dog's liver can't. It takes a dog twice as long to detoxify theobromine as a human.

When you take medicine that needs to be detoxified by your liver, a POTENTIALLY DEADLY ACCUMULATION can happen whenever:

- You take too much medicine at a time or take it too frequently for your liver enzymes to keep up with it.
- Your original quota of liver enzymes is not efficient or fast enough to keep up with the medicine coming in.
- Your liver is damaged, leaving you with fewer liver enzymes.
- You are taking ANOTHER MEDICINE that needs the **exact same liver enzymes to detoxify it,** creating a bottleneck.

When you add another medicine that needs the same liver enzymes as one you are already taking, it's like blocking off your funnel.

- Select several marbles, add them to each of your funnels and then pour water into each funnel. What happens to how fast the water flows out?

- Add a few more marbles and then pour some more water. How fast does the water flow out now?
- As you added more marbles, what happened to the water level in the funnel when you poured in more colored water?

The more marbles you add to the funnel, the less water can flow through and out, causing the water level to rise. If you add enough marbles it will cause an overflow.

You can see a video demonstration of this at www.AskDrLouise.com.

When two (or more) medicines that require the same liver enzymes for detoxification are taken at the same time, the concentration of the those medicines in your body will usually rise.

If you start out with a smaller funnel it will take less medicine to cause a serious backlog, accumulation, and toxicity.

Even if you start out with a larger funnel, if you add marbles (medicines) to it, it will become more like the smaller funnel, and the amount of medicine in your body will increase.

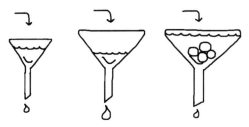

Figure 14. When Medicines Use the Same Liver Enzymes

This can cause a significant increase in blood concentration, leading to side effects, toxicity and even death.

If there can be significant variations between your liver enzymes and someone else's, what about the difference between the enzymes in your liver, and those of your dog or cat?

Your dog's liver doesn't have the same set of liver enzymes that you (as a human) have. Your enzymes help you to safely detoxify theobromine.

Many medicines are removed from your body by your kidneys and sent directly into your urine. Other medicines have to be changed first BEFORE they can be removed.

This process of change is called detoxification, biotransformation, or metabolism and is carried out by your own liver enzymes.

Metabolism changes the shape of a medicine from an active form able to bind to its receptor to an inactive form called a metabolite.

Changing the shape of a medicine through metabolism usually prevents it from binding to its target receptor and helps it to be eliminated by your kidneys.

Some medicines collect in your gall bladder and then are secreted into your small intestine where they move through your intestinal tract and are eliminated in your feces.

How Does a Medicine Get OUT of Your Body?

Medicines are removed or eliminated from your body in one of two ways:

1. Dissolved in your urine
2. Excreted in your feces

Nearly all medicines leave your body by being transported from your bloodstream to your urine through your kidneys and then eliminated as you urinate. The other important way your body removes medicine is through your intestine as you defecate.

Removing a medicine directly out of your bloodstream will make it stop working by moving it OUT of your body so that it can't bind to its target receptor.

Medicines which have already been "deactivated" through transformation or metabolism to an inactive form by your liver enzymes will continue to circulate in your bloodstream until they are physically removed by your kidneys.

Although the transformed medicine is still in your bloodstream for a little while, once it has been made inactive it stops being able to bind to its target receptor and its effect will fade away.

- The ability of your body to detoxify and eliminate medicine is the most critically important part of being able to take medicine safely.

- When too much medicine is taken IN for your body to detoxify and move OUT, the excess can build up to dangerous levels.

- Your kidneys and liver have important roles in detoxifying and eliminating medicines from your body.

- By age 75, you lose nearly 40% of your ability to remove some medicines from your body, which can cause problems with taking medicine safely.

- Liver enzymes are critically important in detoxifying and removing many medicines and poisons from your body.

- Your liver is responsible for detoxifying medicine by changing its shape so it no longer fits on or can bind to its receptor. Once this happens, the medicine stops working and its effect will fade away.

- Your liver enzymes cannot be in two places at once, or attach to more than one medicine at the same time.

- When you take two medicines that use the same liver enzymes for removal, one or both of them can "back up", causing increased and potentially toxic concentrations in your body.

- Removing a medicine directly out of your bloodstream makes it stop working by moving it OUT of your body so that it can't bind to its target receptor.

- The main reason why dogs can't eat chocolate is because a dog's liver enzymes are different than ours. Our liver can easily detoxify theobromine, while a dog's liver can't.

Notes

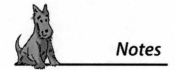

Notes

PART III

How *YOU* Can Take Medicine Safely

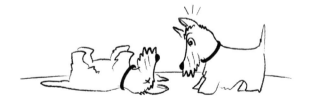

Taking Medicine Safely: The "3 Ds"

7

Most of us can remember the "3 R"s of school:

Reading,

        wRiting, and

                aRithmatic.

Our years in grade school and high school were originally designed to give us these three basic skills: reading, writing and doing basic math. When we graduated, we were expected to be able to read and write in American English, add and subtract groups of numbers, and use multiplication and division to calculate percentages, such as the percent off on a sale, or the % of sales tax owed.

Imagine yourself winning an all-expenses paid 2-week stay at a lovely tropical resort and world-class spa on a white sandy beach. Included in this dream getaway is free travel to and from the resort and a $1000 shopping spree to purchase beach wear before you leave. The only catch is that you need to leave immediately.

Barely 24 hours later, you take your seat in the first class cabin of a Boeing 737 headed for your "vacation of a lifetime". A vintage Land Rover from the resort picks you up at the airport, the smiling driver stowing your new luggage as you climb into the back seat for the last leg of your journey.

Your driver doesn't say much, but you don't notice it because you are distracted by brilliantly colored birds sitting among huge green fronds and the intoxicating fragrance of a warm breeze sweetly scented with exotic flowers.

Just over an hour later, you pull up to the front entrance of your destination resort, collect your bag from the driver and walk into the lobby feeling ready for some relaxation and sightseeing. After greeting the clerk at the front desk to check in, you realize something odd. Your hostess doesn't speak a word of English. In fact, NO ONE in the facility SPEAKS OR UNDERSTANDS A WORD OF ENGLISH!

Because you had to leave for your vacation so quickly, you didn't have time to learn more than a couple of words in the language they are speaking to you.

Unless you learn more words quickly or locate a translator it will be very difficult to take full advantage of your vacation. You'll need to acquire some basic vocabulary in this new language in order to understand the directions to restaurants recommended by your hosts, where the best beach spots are, even how to find a bathroom.

Until you find a way to understand the native language, you'll be missing many opportunities to fully enjoy your good fortune.

Today there is an enormous amount of information available to you about medicines. Newspapers, magazines, and the Internet provide a flood of articles discussing various medicines along with food supplements and herbal products.

You'll find testimonials from people just like you achieving amazing results from products available for immediate purchase. You'll see other articles proclaiming prescription medicines to be a dangerous scam promoted by pharmaceutical manufacturers, then promoting their particular "natural" product, insisting that BECAUSE it comes from "nature" it MUST be safer and more effective than any prescription medicine.

From my three decades of experience as a pharmacist and medication specialist, **prescription and non-prescription medicines are not always dangerous, and "natural" products are not always safe.**

In order to take your medicines safely you MUST know certain basic things about each of the medicines, supplements and herbal products that you (or your loved ones) are taking. I call these basics the "3 Ds".

The "3 Ds" of Taking Medicine Safely
1. **Drug: WHAT you are taking**
2. **Dose: HOW you should take it
   (HOW MUCH and HOW OFTEN)**
3. **Diagnosis: WHY you are taking it**

Knowing these three essentials is VITAL in order for you and your loved ones to take your medicines and supplements safely!

- The single MOST POWERFUL way to take your medicine safely is to keep a list of all your current medicines, and show it to all of your medical providers every single time you get medical care.

- Prescription and non-prescription medicines are NOT always dangerous, and "natural" products are not always safe.

- Your current medication list should include each of the "3 Ds" are for every medicine and supplement you take.

- Knowing WHAT, WHY, HOW MUCH and HOW OFTEN you take each of your medicines is what doctors and medical providers want ALL their patients to know about their medicines.

- The "3 Ds" of taking medicine safely are:

  1. The Drug: WHAT you are taking

  2. The Dose: HOW you should take it (HOW MUCH and HOW OFTEN)

  3. The Diagnosis: WHY you are taking it

Notes

8

The First "D": The Drug (WHAT)

One Saturday morning I was working at the pharmacy and the phone rang. It was a new prescription called in from an urgent care clinic 3 blocks from our store. As I finished taking down the phoned in prescription for an antibiotic, the customer came in looking for it. She waited patiently while we filled the prescription.

I walked over to her with the vial in my left hand, and began to explain, "Your doctor has given you an antibiotic to take, called..." But when I gave her the name of the medicine, she jumped me.

"No, NO! That's not what I wanted!"

"Uh, excuse me...?" I asked, puzzled by her outburst.

"I DON'T want that! I have to get something ELSE!"

"Okaaay..." I tried calming her down. "And that's because...?"

"I've had THAT ONE before and it gave me a terribly awful rash. I just CAN'T take that stuff!"

"Okay, okay, but ma'am, I'm a little confused. This IS what the doctor called in for you this morning. You're saying that you're allergic to this medicine, but the doctor still called it in?"

"Well, not exactly... I felt so sick this morning, and I had such burning when I went pee, I just headed straight down to the urgent clinic. I usually bring my list of medicines with me but I was so uncomfortable, I didn't think about it. I was in such pain, I know I meant to tell them, but maybe I didn't."

"You're SURE that this is the same stuff that you took when you got the rash?"

"Oh, yes. I recognize that name."

"Okay, then. I'll need to call the urgent clinic back and talk to the doctor about this."

"Oh, no, that's okay. I'll stop by my house and get the list and then go back. I've got other allergies on it that I forgot to tell them about."

"All right, then. I'll add this antibiotic to your list of allergies in your records so we'll be able to catch it if this comes up again."

"Thanks. I'll stop by later. I just WISH I'd gone back for that stupid list!"

My patient had rushed out to see the doctor at the urgent clinic without bringing her list of medicines and allergies with her, thinking she'd remember to tell them everything she was allergic to during the visit.

In her discomfort she was so distracted she completely forgot to mention her recent allergic experience to the doctor treating her bladder infection. Luckily, she recognized the name of a medicine she was allergic to in time to avoid another serious allergic reaction.

Knowing the name of each of the medicines that you take is vitally important.

To make it even more confusing, some medicines have *more than one name!* All prescription medicines start out with both a brand name and a generic name. A brand name is the name chosen by the drug manufacturer for marketing purposes.

> The generic name is the official name of the compound, which is the same name used for it all over the world, no matter if it's sold as a brand name product or as a generic.
>
> A medicine's generic name doesn't change.

When the patent protection for a brand name drug runs out, it can be sold as a generic medicine at a lower cost. Compared to the generic name, a brand name is shorter, simpler, easier to pronounce and much easier to spell.

Because the brand name of a new medicine is easier to pronounce and spell than its generic name, many doctors and pharmacists will use the brand name when talking about a medicine.

Even after a medication becomes available as a generic product, many doctors and nurses continue to refer to it by the original name they learned for it, which may not be the name of the medicine on your prescription label.

If you don't recognize both the brand and the generic names of the medicines you are taking, you could get confused if they are used interchangeably. You could even end up with a bottle of each, taking BOTH of them *without realizing that they are the same thing!*

To minimize the risk of getting a dangerous double dose of your medicine, ask your doctor or pharmacist to tell you both the brand and generic names of all your prescription and non-prescription medicines.

When a prescription medicine becomes a non-prescription product, a different brand name may be used to market it, although the generic name stays the same.

Some examples of brand names that have gone from prescription to non-prescription include naproxen, ibuprofen and loperamide.

Naprosyn® is the brand name of naproxen as a prescription medicine. Aleve® is the brand name for the non-prescription form of naproxen. Naproxen as a generic is available both as a prescription and a non-prescription pain reliever.

Imodium® is the brand name of a prescription anti-diarrheal called loperamide. Imodium-AD® is its brand name as a non-prescription medicine. Loperamide is available as a generic in both prescription and non-prescription products.

Motrin® is a brand name of the prescription medication ibuprofen. Generic ibuprofen is available as both a prescription and non-prescription pain reliever. Advil® and Motrin-IB® are examples of brand names of non-prescription ibuprofen.

Knowing the names of each of your medicines, both brand and generic, can help you avoid taking the same medicine twice under two different names. *If you are not sure, please ASK!*

REMEMBER

- Know the names of all the medicines you take.

- Brand names are easier to pronounce and spell than generic names. Medical providers often use the original brand name when talking about a medicine, even after the medicine is available as a generic product.

- Know the brand AND generic name of any medicine you are allergic to.

- When a prescription medicine becomes a non-prescription product, a different brand name may be used to market it, although the generic name will stay the same.

- Knowing the brand and generic names of each of your medicines helps you avoid accidentally taking the same medicine twice, both as the brand name and the generic.

Notes

9

The Second "D": The Dose (HOW and HOW MUCH)

Doctor: "How did those suppositories I gave you work?"

Patient: "Not so good, Doc. I tried one but boy, it has some sharp edges. I had to quit before I cut myself!"

Doctor: "Ah...did you unwrap it first?"

Patient: "Huh?"

A woman complained to her doctor about the pain patch he gave her. "It just doesn't work for me".

When he asked her how she was using it, she explained, "It doesn't stick very well, so I use tape to keep it on."

Further inspection showed that she had never peeled off the clear plastic backing before she put it on. The medicine had never even come in contact with her skin.

It worked much better for her when she peeled off the backing before applying it!

Knowing how to take your medicines, how much to take, and how often to take them can be the difference between a good result and side effects or life-threatening toxicity.

Knowing HOW MUCH medicine to take is very important, because getting TOO MUCH of it can be very dangerous.

There are many medicines that are available both WITH and WITHOUT a prescription. It's not always easy to detect this because medicines are often marketed under one brand name as a prescription and a different one as a non-prescription (over-the-counter, or OTC for short) product.

It's not unusual to receive a prescription medicine containing the same ingredients as an over-the-counter remedy.

To avoid accidental duplication, always ask your doctor or pharmacist before taking any non-prescription medicine.

How much is TOO MUCH Medicine?

Some medicines are very safe when used appropriately, but become very dangerous when too much is taken. One example of this is acetaminophen.

Acetaminophen is a very safe medicine when taken in small amounts. Taking too much Tylenol® or acetaminophen can seriously harm your liver, causing health problems and even organ failure requiring a liver transplant to stay alive.

How much is too much Tylenol® or acetaminophen?

For a healthy adult, the Food and Drug Administration (FDA) recommends a maximum of 4000 mg per day of acetaminophen, the amount in 8 tablets of Extra Strength Tylenol® 500mg.

Due to increasing reports about liver damage from excess acetaminophen, the FDA recently increased their efforts to require new warnings on the label of all products containing acetaminophen to emphasize the risk of liver injury when taking more than 4000mg in a 24-hour period.

Most people who develop liver failure from taking too much acetaminophen never realize they are in danger until it is too late and their liver is already damaged. The popularity of acetaminophen with pharmaceutical manufacturers is a big part of the problem.

Acetaminophen is an active ingredient in hundreds of non-prescription medicines, including ones marketed for allergies, sinus problems, cough, cold and flu symptoms, even problems sleeping.

In 2005, consumers in the United States purchased more than 17 billion doses of non-prescription products containing acetaminophen.

Non-prescription medicines are not the only source of acetaminophen. It also lurks in widely prescribed pain medicines like Vicodin® and Percocet®.

The combination of hydrocodone and acetaminophen has been the most frequently dispensed prescription medicine in the United States every year since 1997, under the brand names Vicodin®, Lortab®, Anexia®, Norco® and their generic equivalents.

How can you protect yourself from getting too much acetaminophen?

You can avoid liver failure from too much acetaminophen by paying careful attention to exactly how much Tylenol® or acetaminophen you take and never taking more than is recommended.

Check the list of ingredients of every medicine you take to make sure you don't exceed the maximum recommended amount of acetaminophen of 4000mg daily.

On prescription labels acetaminophen is often shortened to the abbreviation APAP or ACET.

The FDA is working with the pharmaceutical manufacturing industry to limit the amount of acetaminophen in each tablet of prescription pain relievers to a maximum of 325 mg per tablet.

Acetaminophen is sold as drops, syrup, and chewable tablets for children, regular, extra strength and extended release for adults, and combined with hydrocodone or oxycodone in prescription painkillers.

Ask your pharmacist or doctor about the amount of acetaminophen in the medicines you are currently taking to avoid exceeding the maximum amount that is considered safe for you.

HOW MUCH is too much of an herbal product or food supplement?

Many people believe that compounds extracted from natural sources are perfectly safe for you no matter how much of them you use. Unfortunately, this is not completely true.

Although herbal remedies and food supplements may have fewer side effects than prescription medicine, people who take extra doses in the belief that those compounds "can't harm you because they're natural" are making a dangerous assumption.

One of the most potent heart medicines ever developed is called digoxin or digitalis, originally given as a tea made from the foxglove plant. Other powerful and potentially toxic medications are colchicine and quinine which were originally extracted from plants, and Botox®, also known as botulinum toxin. Poisons such as arsenic, mercury compounds, and strychnine also originate from natural sources.

When it comes to medicines, herbal products and food supplements, more is not necessarily better. Instead, taking more can be toxic, even lethal.

One of the reasons acetaminophen is safe in small doses yet lethal in large doses is how it is eliminated from the body.

Acetaminophen is detoxified by several groups of liver enzymes. Most of the time, the particular enzymes responsible for detoxifying acetaminophen for you do their job with no problems.

However, if your liver is forced to detoxify a large amount of acetaminophen the enzymes responsible for safe removal become overwhelmed, leaving the excess to be shunted down another pathway, like opening another check-out line in a busy grocery store.

The liver enzymes used by the alternative pathway change the excess acetaminophen into a different shape. The final result is a deadly molecule that attaches to a liver cell, killing it.

If you consume excess acetaminophen day after day, eventually YOU WILL DESTROY YOUR LIVER.

If you swallowed the contents of an entire bottle of adult strength acetaminophen all at once, enough killer molecules could be created to completely wipe out or KILL all of the cells in your liver.

If an overdose of acetaminophen is discovered in time, a rescue medicine called acetylcysteine could save your liver from destruction. Acetylcysteine binds directly to the killer molecule produced by the excess acetaminophen, acting to shield your liver cells.

- How much and how often you take your medicine can be the difference between a good result and side effects or life-threatening toxicity.

- When it comes to medicines, herbal products and food supplements, more is not necessarily better. Instead, more can be dangerously toxic.

- Taking excess amounts of herbal remedies and food supplements in the belief that they "can't be harmful because they are natural" is a dangerous assumption.

- Some prescription-only medicines are now available without a prescription, but not always under the original brand name. This can cause confusion and accidental overdose.

- The Food and Drug Administration (FDA) recommends a maximum of 4000 mg per day of acetaminophen for most healthy adults.

- If you consume excess acetaminophen day after day, eventually you will damage your liver cells. Most of the people who develop liver failure from taking too much acetaminophen never realize they are in danger until it is too late and their liver is permanently damaged.

- Non-prescription medicines are not the only source of acetaminophen. It also lurks in popular prescription pain medicines such as Vicodin®, abbreviated on the label as ACET or APAP.

Notes

10

The Third "D": The Diagnosis (WHY)

Seeing Linda in my clinic for the first time, I asked her, "Are you taking any herbal products, or any food supplements?" Linda, like many of my patients, said, "Yes, I am." And she gave me the name of an herbal supplement she was currently taking.

When I asked her, "What are you taking it for?" she shrugged and offered, " I'd like to have more energy. My neighbor swears this stuff works."

I followed up my question with another one: "OK, then, is it working for you?"

"Uh, I'm not sure," she mumbled.

"Linda, if you don't know what it's for, how will you know if it is working?"

If you don't know where you are going, how will you know when you get there? **If you don't know what a drug or herb or supplement is supposed to do, how will you know if it's working?**

Bob had an irregular heartbeat that would occasionally cause him trouble. Out of the blue, his heart would suddenly start racing, and when it did, he had trouble catching his breath.

He went to see his heart doctor for that, and the doctor gave him a prescription medicine to take for his "racing heart". He had just started that medicine when a couple of days later, he had another spell of heart palpitations.

Because it was the weekend, he went to the Emergency department of a local hospital. The doctor in the ER gave him another medicine for his heart, so he filled that as well.

The new heart medicine stopped his episodes of "racing heart", but made him feel tired and sluggish. He didn't have any more problems catching his breath, but he was tired all the time. He felt too "wiped out" to even walk to the mailbox at the end of his driveway.

At our clinic 2 weeks later, Bob mentioned that he had started two new medicines. His heart rate, which had been between 80 and 90 beats per minute, had dropped down to 54 beats per minute. No wonder he felt so tired!

The ER doctor had intended to REPLACE his "old" medicine with the new one, not have him ADD it to his original one. Once he stopped the original medicine he felt much, much better.

WHY are you taking each of your medicines?
Knowing WHY you are taking each of your medicines will help you understand what each medicine is supposed to do for you.

Sometimes your doctor intends to give you another medicine to take in addition to what your are currently taking in order to bring your blood pressure or blood sugar under better control.

Whenever your doctor gives you a new medicine, always ask WHY you are taking it and what reaction to expect.

Be sure to ask your doctor, "Is this new medicine supposed to REPLACE something I'm already taking, or are you ADDING it to my other medicines?"

If you ADD a new medicine to your other ones without STOPPING the "old" one that your doctor is replacing, you can experience unwanted side effects, especially dizziness or drowsiness. You could also faint or fall, causing bruising, broken bones, or a head injury.

Many medicines can do more than one thing and are prescribed for more than one reason. This can be very helpful, because instead of having to take two different medicines, you may only need to take one.

Knowing why you are taking each of your prescription medications and what each pill is for will make it much easier for your doctors to adjust your medicine to do the very best job for you.

If you know what each of your medicines are for, when you ask your pharmacist about what you can safely take for your cough or cold, he or she will have the information they need to best advise you. Your pharmacist is trained to help you choose products to ease your misery without interfering with your prescription medicines.

Knowing WHY you are taking your medicine can help you avoid getting the wrong drug by accident, especially when taking it for the first time.

Doctors are only human, and computers are making prescriptions more legible but not infallible. With so many medicines having similar sounding names and spellings it's possible to end up getting a prescription for a very different medicine than what your doctor intended for you.

Whenever you fill a new prescription, if you know WHY you are taking it, you can double-check with your pharmacist that your new medicine is actually used for that purpose.

I was in the middle of explaining about a new medicine to George when he interrupted me, asking, "Are you SURE this is the right stuff? My doctor told me this was supposed to be for my heart, and you're saying it's for depression."

"That's possible, George." I responded. "Let's check that out. I'll go pull the original prescription we received from your doctor, okay?"

When I found the original prescription, an error HAD been made, but it was by US. We had filled George's prescription with fluoxetine 20mg one daily, an antidepressant, instead of with furosemide 20mg one daily, for congestive heart failure.

If George hadn't spoken up, he could easily have ended up in the hospital!

REMEMBER

- If you don't know what a medicine, supplement, or herbal product is supposed to do, how will you know if it's working?

- Knowing WHY you are taking each of your medicines helps you understand what each medicine is supposed to do for you.

- Knowing WHY you are given a new medicine allows you to clarify with your doctor whether it's IN ADDITION to what you already take, or IN PLACE of it.

- If you know what each of your medicines are for, when you ask your pharmacist about what you can safely take for your cough or cold, he or she will have the information they need to best advise you.

- Knowing WHY you are taking your medicine can help you avoid getting the wrong drug by accident.

Notes

Notes

5 Key Strategies For Protecting You and Your Loved Ones From The Dangers of Drug Therapy

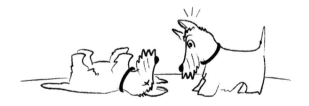

11

Keep A List

Make a list of ALL your medications, including every prescription and non-prescription medicine, any vitamins, herbal remedies and any supplements.

Be sure to include WHY you are taking each one, keep it up to date and show it to ALL of your medical providers every time you receive any medical or dental care.

The most important thing you can do to take your medicine safely is to keep a current list of all your medicines and take it with you to EVERY medical and dental appointment.

When Making Your Medication List:
- Include EVERY medicine, vitamin, supplement and herbal product you are CURRENTLY taking.
- List any allergies or adverse reactions you've experienced.

- **Update your list frequently and show it to ALL of your medical providers at EVERY visit.**

This one habit will get you far, far better medical care than if you leave it completely up to an overworked health care team to keep track of what medicines you are taking.

If the doctors, dentists, chiropractors, nurses and pharmacists who care for you don't know EXACTLY what you are taking and what you have had problems with in the past, they are working blind. They cannot do their best for you if they're missing this vitally important information.

Estelle, one of my older patients had a painful bladder infection, and was prescribed an antibiotic by her urologist.

On the second day of taking it, she noticed itchy, fiery red patches on her arms and trunk.

When I asked her what medicine she had been taking, she said, "The doctor gave me Bactrim®. See? It's right on my the medicine bottle." And it was.

"Have you ever taken any sulfa drugs before?" I asked her.

"Oh, yes, last winter while I was in San Diego, I was given Septra® for a sinus infection. It made me puff up like, JUST LIKE THIS! They told me not to take any more sulfa drugs. But Bactrim® isn't a sulfa drug, is it?"

"I'm afraid so. Bactrim® and Septra® are BOTH sulfa drugs. I don't see either of them on our list of your allergies. Did you tell the urology clinic that you're allergic to sulfa?"

"No", she answered, with a big sigh. "I guess I need to tell them, so there isn't a next time."

"I'll add this to our records. But you need another antibiotic, and something for the itching and swelling. I think the doctor will want to see you right away."

Why is making a medication list and showing it to your doctor so critically important?

Keeping a current list of all your medicine and allergies helps show your doctors which medicines you've already had that gave you problems, either from an allergic reaction or other undesirable response.

This warns your medical providers and minimizes the chance that you'll be given one of those medicines again.

 If your medical professional isn't aware of what has given you a bad reaction in the past, you could end up taking that medicine again, causing you inconvenience, discomfort or a life-threatening reaction.

Your list should always include why you are taking each medicine. Your doctor is best able to choose the best treatment for you and avoid giving you medicines that could interact with what you're already taking if he or she is aware of the reason you're taking each of your medicines, vitamin and supplements.

It's also very helpful to include the name of the medical provider prescribing each of the medicines on your list.

Many doctors use computerized record keeping systems for your medical information, but they don't always get records sent to them from all the other providers that you see. This is especially true if your visit to the other doctor was a recent one.

If your medical provider knows who else is taking care of you, if they have a question or a concern about your medicine, they'll know whom to call in order to consult with them.

Another important detail that should be on your list is the ACTUAL dose you are taking. This includes the size of the tablet or capsule, and how frequently you are taking it.

Keeping a current list of your medicines prevents a LOT of wasted time and guesswork for medical professionals taking care of you.

Hospitals are now required to make a good faith effort to reconstruct the list of medicines of each patient who is admitted to their facility.

If you don't present a medication list to them, they will be forced to track down and contact your primary care physician and your pharmacy to verify as best as they can what your current medications consist of.

This process is called medication reconciliation, and is one of the most important ways you can help prevent medication errors during a hospitalization.

If you have had a medication adjusted from seeing a specialist or during a hospital stay, your doctor may not be aware of it.

The dose that you are taking NOW may not be what is listed in your chart or match the label directions of your current prescription.

If you are a patient at a hospital, a new medication list is also required when you are discharged, including any new medicines that the hospital physicians have started during the course of your hospital stay.

If you have your medicine list from BEFORE you were in the hospital, you can compare your BEFORE list with any changes during your hospital stay and keep yourself on track.

The main reason hospitals are now required to collect and verify current medication lists for their patients is because **some of the most common, dangerous, yet PREVENTABLE medicine errors happen during hospitalizations.**

Mistakes or misunderstandings in your medicine after being released from the hospital are commonplace and can send you back to the hospital, or worse, to the morgue!

Making and keeping a list of your medicines will make it much easier for you to use a pill box effectively. You can ensure that all of your regular medications are set up for each day of the week as you fill each compartment from your list.

To help get you started using a pill box for the first time, I have included a pill box worksheet form that can double as a medication list for you. You can also download a full size version at my website, at www.AskDrLouise.com/products.

When your medicines change, now you can update your medication list easily. An updatable version of my pill box worksheet is now available. To get your free copy of Dr. Louise's Updatable Pill Box Worksheet go to www.AskDrLouise.com/products.

- Make a list of EVERY medicine, vitamin, supplement and herbal product you're CURRENTLY taking.

- Include any allergies or adverse reactions to medications that you've experienced.

- Update your medicine list whenever you start a new one or change any of your medicines.

- Take your list to EVERY medical and dental visit, and show it to ALL your medical and dental providers, including any hospital or medical facilities.

- When you are discharged from a medical facility, compare the list of medicines in your printed discharge instructions to your previous list or medicines you were taking before your hospital stay and clarify any discrepancies.

Notes

12

Use A Pill Box

Use a pill box for your medicine with compartments for each day of the week.

A pill box decreases the risk of either running completely out of your pills or accidently taking a "double dose", turning an innocent mistake into a life-threatening situation.

One of the most useful tools I recommend to help you take your medicine safely is a pill box or pill minder.

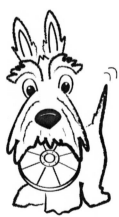

We're all very busy, and our lives are punctuated with interruptions from phones, visitors and other commitments.

It's very easy to get distracted and forget to take your medicine or forget that you've ALREADY taken your medicine!

For the past 18 years I have been taking care of people who take blood thinners. With some medicines if you miss a day taking it here and there it doesn't matter. Blood thinner medicines need to be taken as consistently as possible because forgetting to take your medicine can trigger a stroke or blood clot.

Too much blood thinner medicine is also dangerous. Inadvertently taking an extra dose of blood thinner because you weren't aware that you had already taken it can cause serious, life-threatening bleeding.

I recommend using a pill box to all my patients who take any kind of heart medicines or blood thinners because it reduces the risk of taking too much or too little medicine.

Pill boxes come in many shapes; some have only one compartment for each day of the week, while others have 3 or 4 compartments for each day. Most pharmacies have a good selection and can help you choose the one that fits you the best.

If you have any vitamins, calcium, or potassium supplements you will probably need a pill box with larger sized compartments in order to fit all your pills into it.

4 Great Reasons To Use A Pill Box:

1. **No More Guessing**

   You don't have to guess if you have already taken your medicine. If you flip open today's compartment and the pill is still there, you haven't taken it yet. If the pill is gone, then you can reassure yourself that you took it.

2. **More Timely Refills**

   When you are filling your pill box for the next week ahead, if you don't have enough medicine to completely fill all the compartments for the week, you're reminded to contact your pharmacy for a refill, giving them days of warning instead of calling only after you've taken the very last pill in your medicine bottle.

3. **More Compact When Traveling**

   A pill box usually takes up less space than the full size bottles of medicine, vitamins and supplements you may take. If you misplace a pill box while on a trip you'll still have the rest of your medicines safe at home.

4. **Family or Caregivers Can Help You**

   As we age, we may get confused and mix up our medicines. Using a pill box allows a caregiver or family member to help us out, either by double-checking the compartments to make sure that they are correctly filled up, or by assisting with the filling process.

Some pharmacies are able to provide your medicines already organized by day of the week in "bubble-packs" or "compliance packaging". The medicine is pre-loaded in flat cards with individual compartments for each day of the week similar to a blister-pack.

You may also be able to have it delivered to your residence. Ask your doctor or pharmacist about the availability of this service.

Loading a pill box for the first time can be overwhelming. The most important thing is to line up your bottles of medicine and fill each of the daily compartments, using one medicine bottle at a time.

Make sure to fill all the compartments for the week before going to the next bottle of medicine. When I finish putting all of a particular medicine into the pill box, I flip the prescription bottle over onto its top to show that I am done with it.

I find that it's much easier to fill a pill box quickly, correctly, and completely if you have a little help. To do this, I developed a worksheet to help me get it right. It's in the appendix of the back of this book, or you can download a full-size PDF of Dr. Louise's Pill Box Worksheet free from my website at www.AskDrLouise.com/products.

When filling your pill box it's important to use a current medication list. To help you do that, an updatable version of my pill box worksheet is now available. To get your free copy of Dr. Louise's Updatable Pill Box Worksheet go to www.AskDrLouise.com/products.

REMEMBER

- Using a pill box with compartments for each day of the week decreases the risk of either running completely out of your pills or taking an extra dose by accident.

- You can verify if you have taken your pills for the day by checking that day's compartment of your pill box. If the pill is gone, you can reassure yourself that you have already taken it.

- With a pill box, you're reminded to contact your pharmacy for a refill days before you actually run out of your medicine.

- Using a pill box allows a caregiver or family member to help out by either double-checking each compartment to make sure that they are correctly filled up or by loading it themselves.

- A pill box usually takes up less space when traveling than the full size bottles of medicine, vitamins and supplements that you take.

- If your pill box gets lost or left behind on a trip, you'll still have the rest of your medicines safe at home.

- Some pharmacies are able to provide medicines already organized by day of the week in blister-pack cards and even deliver them to your residence.

Notes

13

Be A
Squeaky Wheel

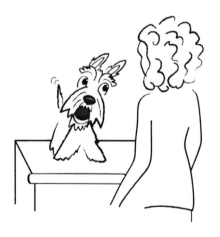

Speak up if you feel crummy after having a medicine changed or adjusted, especially if it's new to you.

Tell your doctor if you have stopped taking any of your medicines, and why, so you can work together to find another way to treat your medical condition.

When I asked Gladys, an elderly patient of mine, how things were going with her, she said, "Fine, I guess. But my arthritis is getting worse, and it's slowing me down. I really shouldn't complain...but it's no fun getting older."

I looked over her medical chart and asked her, "Have you started any new medicines in the last few months?"

"Well, yes. My heart doctor started me on one, oh, almost 2 months ago now, for my cholesterol."

"When did you notice your arthritis getting worse?"

"Only since the last couple of months. Why, do you think it might have something to do with it?"

"I think you should call your heart doctor and tell him about it right away. If you don't speak up, how is he going to know you're having problems?"

When I saw Gladys again, three months later, she came right up to me and said, "Dr. Louise, thank you for having me call my doctor on that medicine. He had me stop it and I was feeling like my old self in just a few days. When I think of what I put up with...and it wasn't my arthritis at all!"

Gladys' physician was someone I knew as a very competent and caring physician. *He was NOT, however, a mind reader!*

When a doctor prescribes a medicine to you, "no news is good news". Unless a doctor hears otherwise, he or she will assume that things are going well for you on the medicine.

REMEMBER

If you suspect you could be experiencing side effects from a medicine, you NEED to contact your doctor and tell him or her about it!

I've been shocked and dismayed many times in my career when I learn about the YEARS of misery some people have endured, all because they assume that nothing can be done. **They suffer in silence, believing that it's just old age creeping up on them or that telling their doctor about any discomfort would be useless complaining.**

Some restless souls are hyper-vigilant, constantly on the phone to their doctor about their symptoms and insisting on yet another medicine. I have encountered far, far more folks who have suffered silently, **convinced that because their doctor prescribed it, they must endure it, no matter how awful it makes them feel.**

That's *rubbish!*

When it comes to reactions to medicines, you are unique. NO medicine works the same on everyone!

You are unique in the number and type of medicine receptors you have in your body. **There is no way to predict whether a particular medicine will work as expected, not work at all, or give you an unusual, idiosyncratic or completely opposite reaction.**

If you look at the list of possible side effects included with every prescription dispensed by your pharmacy, it will give details only on adverse effects already reported by people taking that medicine. Just because a side effect isn't very common doesn't mean it can't happen to you!

If you have quit taking any of your medicines, it's very important to tell your doctor about it, and why you stopped.

Some medicines are much harder to tolerate when given together. Your body is unique in how fast it can detoxify and eliminate medicines, especially when another one is added to the other medicines you already take.

If you don't tell your doctor that you have quit taking your medicine, your condition goes untreated, sometimes leading to serious problems like heart attack, kidney damage, or stroke.

Help your doctor give you the best medical care possible by giving him or her an update of how you are doing when you begin a new prescription medicine.

Without this, they MUST assume that everything is going well with you.

- Speak up if you feel crummy after having a medicine changed or adjusted, especially if it's a new one for you.

- Tell your doctor if you have stopped taking any of your medicines, and why.

- No medicine works the same in everyone. When it comes to reactions to medicines, you are unique.

- Your doctor isn't a mind reader. He or she will assume that things are going well with a new medicine unless you let him or her know otherwise.

- If you don't tell your doctor that you have quit taking your medicine, your condition goes untreated with possibly serious results.

- If you suspect you could be experiencing side effects from a medicine, contact your doctor about it.

- Don't suffer in silence. Be a "squeaky wheel" by speaking up!

Notes

14   Always ASK

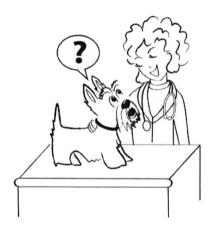

When you start a new medicine, ASK your doctor why you are taking it and what you should expect when taking it.

If you start having problems with any of your medicines, don't be shy. ASK your pharmacist or doctor about it.

If you feel your doctor or pharmacist doesn't listen to you or understand you, find another one.

I'll never forget that Wednesday morning when I took the call from Mrs. Adams. She'd had a question about the patches we'd delivered to her the day before.

"I was sure stumped. I couldn't figure out how to get the patch to stay on. Is it okay to use medical tape? It's the only thing that seems to work."

"Ah, have you peeled the back paper off? There's adhesive on the back of it, just like a Band-Aid®."

"Really? That WOULD be easier. Thank you!"

If you aren't sure how to take a medicine, PLEASE don't stay quiet. ASK your doctor or your pharmacist.

If you are not sure what a new medicine is for or is supposed to do, ASK your doctor.

If you are not sure what to expect when starting a new medicine, ASK your doctor or pharmacist.

If you need to take something for aches, pains, or cough and cold symptoms, ASK your pharmacist. He or she is highly trained in what to recommend that will not interfere with the prescription medicine you are taking.

If you get only one month's supply of medicine at a time and you'd like more, ASK your doctor for a 90-day supply, or have your pharmacist request it for your next refill.

Whenever your doctor gives you on a new medicine, ASK him or her if it will be REPLACING another medicine you are taking or if it is IN ADDITION to the others you already take.

ASK your pharmacist if there are any special conditions that could affect your new medicine:

- Should it be taken on an empty stomach?
- Should it be taken with or without food or milk?
- Are alcoholic beverages safe to drink while taking it?
- Should your new medicine be taken at a certain time of day, such as in the morning or at bedtime?
- Is your medicine supposed to be taken regularly, or just when you have specific symptoms?
- Is your new medicine likely to cause drowsiness or affect your ability to drive a car safely?
- Does this medicine cause sensitivity to the sun? Should you avoid being in direct sunlight, wear sunscreen or cover up?

Always double-check each new bottle of medicine BEFORE you leave the pharmacy by opening the vial and looking at the pills. If they don't look right to you, ASK your pharmacist about it.

If you aren't sure what your new medicine is supposed to do, ASK!

Your pharmacist is an expert on medications, and is trained to answer your questions about your pills. **Pharmacists don't just fill prescriptions; they're the best allies you can possibly have to help you take your medicines safely.**

No other medical professional has the specialized training and experience in recognizing potential problems with medicines and crafting clever solutions to the challenges of drug therapy.

Pharmacists are highly trained in every aspect of how medicines work and how to identify and solve the common and unique problems patients may experience when taking medicine.

Because their training focuses specifically on treatment with medicines, your pharmacist knows medicines in far more detail and depth than most physicians.

Your pharmacist can be your best protection against medication mishaps.

ASK your pharmacist WHENEVER you have a question about your medicine!

If you start having problems with any of your medicines, don't be shy. ASK your pharmacist or doctor about it. If you feel they don't listen to you or understand you, find another medical professional that you feel more comfortable with.

- When starting a new medicine, ASK your doctor why you are taking it and what you should expect from it.

- When starting a new medicine, ASK your doctor if it REPLACES another medicine you are currently taking or is ADDED to it.

- If you start having problems with any of your medicines, don't be shy. ASK your pharmacist or doctor about it.

- If you aren't sure how to take a medicine, ASK your doctor or pharmacist.

- Your pharmacist knows medicines in far more detail and depth than most physicians, and can be your best ally in taking your medicine safely.

- If your pills don't look right to you, ASK your pharmacist to check on it for you.

- If you feel your doctor doesn't listen to or understand you, find another who does.

Notes

15 Don't Share

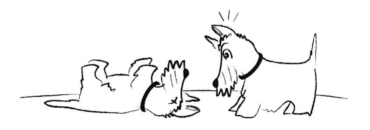

Resist the temptation to try out other people's prescription medicine, and don't offer yours to share.

A medicine that is perfectly safe for YOU could be dangerous when combined with someone else's pills.

As the shrill tones of my fire department emergency pager shrieked in my ears, the red numbers of my digital alarm clock read 02:10 on a Sunday morning in early February. I quickly pulled on the field pants draped over the bedpost at the foot of my bed, followed by a base layer of sports bra and thermal undershirt.

Next over my head came a sweatshirt with NILE FIRE, in bold white capital letters on the back. I was at the back door just finishing putting on my boots, when the dispatcher's calm alto voice announced, "Nile Fire, woman down, age 65, possible seizure, private residence."

A medical emergency, then, not a fire call. As one of only five Emergency Medical Technicians on our small rural fire department, I was going to be needed.

As the officer on call this weekend, I had parked the command rig in my driveway so I didn't have to hustle to our main station nearly two miles away to catch a ride to the incident.

Climbing up into the red Ford 4-wheel-drive club cab pickup truck, I radioed back to fire dispatch, "Nile 5, responding" and eased down my gravel driveway out to the main highway, turning on my emergency lights and siren when I hit the pavement.

I could make out the flashing white and red lights of our aid car just ahead on my left, and slowed down as I approached. One of my guys waved me onto the patient's driveway nearly hidden in the trees. I parked my rig 15 feet behind our ambulance, allowing room to open its big bay doors and load a stretcher.

My clipboard in hand, I found the patient still on the floor, with three firefighters clustered around her and a second woman on a nearby sofa wringing her hands.

After checking that the woman on the floor was indeed the patient and that she was breathing and being taken care of, I focused on getting some history from the lady on the couch. Emily was visiting her sister and had brought with her some weight loss pills prescribed by her physician back in Minnesota. Since they weren't working for her, she offered them to her sister Jeannie to try, saying, "I was just going to have to throw them away."

Jeannie had taken at least one of the pills earlier that evening, and gone to bed about midnight. Emily was awakened an hour later by her sister complaining of heart palpitations and "feeling the world was going to end."

They were debating whether to drive into town to the hospital ER when Jeannie started shivering and shaking all over and couldn't stop. That's when Emily got scared and called 911.

The prescription bottle with Emily's name on it contained Redux®, a weight loss medicine that was pulled off the market in September of that year because of being associated with heart valve problems in otherwise health young people who took it to lose weight.

Jeannie's prescription antidepressant had interacted with the Redux®, precipitating symptoms of feeling her heart racing, anxiety and uncontrollable shaking.

Luckily, Jeannie didn't suffer any permanent problems. But Emily and Jeannie will never forget that harrowing February morning.

When you have a headache, it seems perfectly natural to borrow from your family or friends, "Anyone have some ibuprofen or Tylenol® I can borrow? I have a killer headache and I don't have any with me."

Resist the urge to share your prescription medicines with anyone else, and don't experiment with taking other people's pills.

Remember the two different sized funnels? They show how we can be different in how fast we can detoxify and remove medicines. **What may be a perfectly safe medicine for someone else could be dangerous or even lethal when added to YOUR pills!**

Avoid giving any prescription or non-prescription medicines to your pet without checking first with your veterinarian.

Just as chocolate is deadly to dogs, acetaminophen or Tylenol® is dangerous to cats.

If you're interested in changing your medication or trying something you've seen advertised or heard about, talk with your doctor FIRST about your options. He or she has your medical information and should already have a copy of your current medication list, to advise you on the best medicine for you.

- Resist the temptation to try out other peoples' prescription medicine, and don't offer yours to share.

- Don't share your prescription medicine or give any non-prescription products to your pet without first checking with a veterinarian.

- If you're interested in trying a new medicine, talk with your doctor FIRST before experimenting with someone else's prescription medication.

- What may be a perfectly safe prescription medicine for someone else could be dangerous or even lethal when combined with YOUR pills.

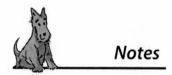

Notes

PART V

25 Ways You Can Avoid Medication Mishaps

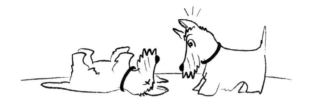

25 Ways You Can Avoid Medication Mishaps

1. Make sure you understand exactly WHAT each of your medicines and supplements is supposed to do.
2. When taking medication, do your best to take it faithfully and only according to your doctor's instructions.
3. MORE is not always better. Don't "double-up" your medicines or supplements.
4. Keep medicines out of reach of children, grandchildren, and pets.
5. Be a squeaky wheel. Speak up if you are having problems with a new medicine.
6. ASK your doctor or pharmacist if you have any questions about your medicine.
7. Let your pharmacist be your ally. He or she has dedicated their career to helping people like you avoid medication mishaps.

8. Using one local pharmacy allows your pharmacist to get to know you and your medicines, where they are in a better position to recognize potential problems and advise you.

9. If you can't understand your doctor or pharmacist, find another.

10. Avoid using mail order pharmacies if you can. Instead, choose a pharmacy where you feel comfortable asking the pharmacists questions, then ASK!

11. Use a pill box, pill minder or "bubble pack" to help you remember to take your medicine.

12. If you suspect you are experiencing side effects from a medicine, contact your doctor and let him or her know about it.

13. If you feel your medical professional doesn't listen to you, find another.

14. 'Fess up. If you haven't been taking your medicine, admit it to your medical provider and tell him or her WHY.

15. If you don't feel very good after starting a new medicine, speak up!

16. Before you take any medication, potion or pill, take just a moment and read the label first, making sure that it is what you think it is.

17. When starting a new herbal product or supplement, use a symptom diary to help you answer the question, "Is it working for me?"

18. Double-check any new bottle of pills by opening it up and taking a look...BEFORE you leave the pharmacy.

19. When buying herbal products, buy ones that list their ingredients "by assay", or the actual amount in each bottle.

20. Update your list of medications whenever you start something new.

21. Include a fourth "D" for each of the medicines on your medicine list: the doctor who prescribed it.

22. Share a current list of ALL your medications, food supplements and herbal products with ALL your medical providers EVERY time you see them.
23. Include any allergies or adverse reactions to medicine in your current medication list.
24. Treat herbals and supplements with respect. Just because they are natural in origin doesn't mean they can't harm you.
25. You are unique. No drug works the same on everyone. If something doesn't seem right, speak up!

References

1. Institute of Medicine of the National Academies, Preventing Medication Errors, National Academies Press, 2007, p 124.
2. Unintentional Drug Poisoning in the United States. Centers for Disease Control and Prevention. July 2010.
    http://www.cdc.gov/HomeandRecreational- Safety/pdf/poison-issue-brief.pdf
    Accessed 1/3/2013.
3. National Ambulatory Medical Care Survey: 2009 Summary tables 18 through 23. Downloaded from www.cdc.gov/hchs/fastats/drugs.htm on 11/19/2012.
4. Miller KB et al. Survey of Commercially Available Chocolate- and Cocoa-Containing Products in the United States. J. Agric.Food Chem. 2009, 57, pages 9169-9180. Downloaded from pubs.acs/org/JAFC on 12/15/2012, with thanks to Kenneth Miller and the Hershey Center for Health and Nutrition.

Appendix
Resources

Pet Poison Centers

Both the Pet Poison Helpline and the ASPCA Animal Poison Information Center have websites which have a LOT of great information about which foods are NOT good to feed your pet and how to "pet-proof" your home.

PLEASE NOTE: The fees stated below are those current at the time of publication.

Pet Poison Helpline
(800) 213-6680
www.petpoisonhelpline.com
$35 fee

ASPCA Animal Poison Information Center

(888) 426-4435

www.aspca.org/pet-care/poison-control/

$65 fee

Some local Poison Centers also provide pet poisoning services for a fee. The national toll-free phone number will connect you directly with the poison center nearest you.

Your local Poison Control Center (United States)
(800) 222-1222

If you suspect your pet has been poisoned, ALWAYS call your veterinarian, a pet poison center, or your local poison center FIRST before giving them anything to encourage vomiting.

Some compounds are caustic and will cause far more damage by being vomited back up than if they were left alone. Your veterinary professional will be able to advise you about when to encourage vomiting.

You may want to keep an unopened bottle of 3% hydrogen peroxide with an oral syringe (it has a wider opening than a standard syringe) next to it in case you are instructed by a veterinary professional or poison center to induce your dog to vomit.

The usual dose is 1ml for every pound your dog weighs. I keep a 20ml oral syringe handy by rubber-banding it to an unopened bottle of household 3% hydrogen peroxide for my Scottish Terriers.

WARNING: Hydrogen peroxide may work VERY FAST and can bleach clothing and carpeting.

Looking for an App to Help You Keep Track of Your Medicines?

Here are some great sources for apps. Keep checking back for updates to their site as they add new options.

Washington State Patient Safety Coalition

www.mymedicinelist.org

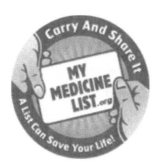

My Medicine List is a campaign to build public awareness toward managing your medicines. Its goal is for every person to maintain an up-to-date list of all their medicines and to share it with all their health providers at every visit.

For iPhone, iPod Touch and Android apps:

www.wapatientsafety.org/my-medicine-list/examples

For downloadable hard copy versions of medication lists:

www.wapatientsafety.org/my-medicine-list/examples

Other Resources For Medication Safety

Food and Drug Administration (FDA)

www.fda.gov/ForConsumers

My Medicine Record is a downloadable file that helps you create your own medication list. It is available at: www.fda.gov/Drugs/ResourcesForYou/ucm079489

FDA Animal Health Information

www.fda.gov/AnimalVeterinary/Resources for You

Important safety alerts including medication errors and your pet and pet food safety.

American Society of Health-Systems Pharmacists (ASHP)

www.safemedicine.com

My Medicine List™ is a downloadable PDF to help you create your own medication list. ASHP also has a drug information searchable database, advice on how to administer medicines, and a pharmacist blog.

National Institutes for Health (NIH)

www.nihseniorhealth.gov/takingmedicinessafely

This website was developed by the National Institute on Aging and the National Library of Medicine. It has a lot of good information about taking medicine safely.

Institute for Safe Medication Practices (ISMP)

www.ismp.org

www.consumermedsafety.org

The ISMP is a nonprofit organization devoted entirely to educating medical professionals and consumers about medication error prevention. They have great articles geared to a general audience and a newsletter at www.consumermedsafety.org.

A percentage from the sale of each book of *Why Dogs Can't Eat Chocolate* will be donated to the Institute for Safe Medicine Practices Foundation to support their important work in making medication prescribing, dispensing and administration safer for all of us.

National Council on Patient Information and Education (NCPIE)

www.talkaboutrx.org

The NCPIE is a non-profit coalition of nearly 100 organizations dedicated to empower consumers to be more informed about and active in decisions about their medicines by stimulating communication between them and their health care professionals.

NCPIE has a great resource to help you make the most of your visit to your physician or health care professional: the **Make Notes and Take Notes** guide, which is a great way to get your questions answered by your medical professional. A full-size version is at *www.talkaboutrx.org/documents/make_notes_bw.pdf*.

Ask Dr Louise

www.AskDrLouise.com

Blog and articles to help you take your medicine safely, with free downloads including **Taking Warfarin Safely** and a Pill Box Worksheet.

Dr. Louise's Pill Box Worksheet is designed to help you use a pill box for the first time or to double check your pill box when done. This free downloadable worksheet has room to count the number of pills in each compartment to help you double-check your accuracy.

There are two different versions of the Pill Box Worksheet: one standard and one updatable, both available *FREE* from www.AskDrLouise.com under Products.

Make Notes & Take Notes

Before, during, and after my doctor's visit

Helpful Steps to Avoid Medication Errors

Before My Doctor's Visit

Date of visit _____

Doctor's name_____
Address _____

Phone _____
Reason for this visit _____
_____

Symptoms/medical problem you are having
_____
_____
_____

How long have you had this problem or symptoms? _____
_____

Questions you want to ask the doctor about this problem or symptoms _____
_____
_____

> **List below all of the prescription and non-prescription (OTC) medicines you are now taking.**

(Show this list to you doctor during your visit)

Prescription Medicines
_____
_____
_____
_____

Over-the-Counter (nonprescription) Medicines and Vitamins / Minerals, Dietary / Herbal Supplements
_____
_____
_____
_____
_____
_____

At the Doctor's Office

Record any diagnosis (name of the problem) your doctor gives you _____
_____
_____
_____

Record the name and phone number of any other doctor that you should see about your medical problem
Name _____
Phone _____

> **Questions to Ask About Prescription Medicines**

(If my doctor prescribes medicine for me, here are some important questions to ask)

1. What is the name of the medicine and what is it for? _____

❑ brand name or the ❑ generic name?

2. How and when do I take it—and for how long? _____

3. What side effects should I expect, and what should I do about them? _____

4. Should I take this medicine on an ❑ empty stomach or ❑ with food?
Is it safe to drink alcohol with this medicine ❑ yes or ❑ no

5. If it's a once-a-day dose, is it best to take it in the ❑ morning or ❑ evening?

6. What foods, drinks, or activities should I avoid while taking this medicine? _____
_____

7. Will this medicine work safely with any other medicines I am taking? ❑ yes ❑ no

8. When should I expect the medicine to begin to work, and how will I know if it is working?
_____

Are there any tests required with this medicine (for example, to check liver or kidney function)?
_____
_____

9. How should I store this medicine?
_____
_____

10. Is there any written information available about the medicine?
❑ yes or ❑ no?
Is it available in large print or a language other than English? ❑ yes or ❑ no?
_____

After My Doctor's Visit

Call your doctor immediately if you are having any problems with your treatment.

Call your doctor or pharmacist if you think you are having troubling side effects with any medicine prescribed or recommended for you.
Pharmacy _____
Phone _____

Record the date and time for any scheduled blood tests, x-rays, or other medical tests ordered by your doctor
Test _____
Phone _____
Testing facility_____

Record the date and time of your next doctor's visit _____

> **Keep up to date**
> **Use 1 sheet for each doctor you visit**

EDUCATE *before*
YOU MEDICATE

National Council on Patient Information and Education (NCPIE)
200-A Monroe Street, Suite 212
Rockville, MD 20840
(301) 340-3940
www.talkaboutrx.org

Reprinted by gracious permission of the NCPIE

Ask Dr. Louise Medication List / Pill Box Worksheet

Start Here: **Name:** _____ **DOB:** _____

Use this form to help you fill your pill box every week:

1. List ALL of your allergies, medications and supplements in the boxes
2. Show this list to ALL of your medical care providers
3. Update this list regularly

Allergies/Adverse Reactions:

Drug	What happened?

Medication List and Pill Box Fill Sheet:

Name	Dose	Directions	AM	Noon	PM	Bed	Doctor	Why I'm taking it

Number of pills in each compartment:

Helping You Take Your Medicine Safely™

www.AskDrLouise.com

About the Author

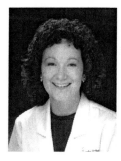

Dr. Louise Achey, Pharm.D, BCPS has practiced pharmacy in hospitals, nursing homes, and community pharmacies for the past 34 years. She teaches medical, pharmacy and physician assistant students, family medicine physicians and also blogs on medication safety and other topics at www.AskDrLouise.com.

A graduate of the School of Pharmacy at Washington State University in 1979, Dr. Louise completed her Doctor of Pharmacy from Idaho State University in 1994 and became specialty certified in Pharmacotherapy in 1997.

She has taught at the College of Pharmacy at Washington State University and is Clinical Assistant Professor of Family Medicine at the University of Washington School of Medicine as well as faculty at the Central Washington Family Medicine Residency Program in Yakima, WA.

Dr. Achey is the author of the newspaper column Ask Dr. Louise and the products **Bladder Bliss** and **Taking Warfarin Safely.** For a presentation or workshop contact her at www.AskDrLouise.com.

About the Artist

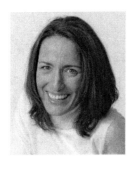

Alece Birnbach is a skilled illustrator, painter and sculptor working as a professional artist for 25 years. Over 100 of her fashionable and fabulous designs appear on products at an array of mid and mass market retailers.

Alece started her career as an art director and then owned an award-winning agency. She applies her knowledge of targeting audiences and building brands in creating the designs for her whimsical characters and collections at www.alecebirnbach.com.

Other Products
by Dr. Louise Achey

Dr. Louise's Pill Box Worksheet
FREE! Helping you take your medicine safely
www.AskDrLouise.com

Bladder Bliss
Natural bladder control without drugs or surgery
www.BladderBliss.com

Taking Warfarin Safely
Staying safe, travel and eating tips when taking warfarin
www.PocketMediGuides.com

Dr. Louise is also available for presentations and workshops on taking your medicine safely.

Contact Dr. Louise Achey at:
louise@AskDrLouise.com
Phone: (509) 658-2570
Fax: (509) 658-2570

CPSIA information can be obtained at www.ICGtesting.com
Printed in the USA
LVOW13*1949190614

390830LV00013B/624/P